TRANSPERSONAL HYPNOSIS

Gateway to Body, Mind, and Spirit

TRANSPERSONAL HYPNOSIS

Gateway to Body, Mind, and Spirit

Edited by

Eric D. Leskowitz, M.D.

CRC Press

Boca Raton   London   New York   Washington, D.C.

Library of Congress Cataloging-in-Publication Data

Transpersonal hypnosis: gateway to body, mind, and spirit / edited by Eric D. Leskowitz
     p. cm.
   Includes bibliographical references and index.
   ISBN 0-8493-2237-5 (alk. paper)
   1. Hypnotism. I. Leskowitz, Eric D.
BF1141.T75 1999
154.7—dc21   97-32274
                                                              CIP

Introduction

The last years of the 20th century in America are witnessing an amazing outgrowth of interest in altered states of consciousness and spirituality. Topics that would normally be discussed *sub rosa*, if at all, have penetrated professional circles in disciplines as widespread as medicine (holistic medicine and spiritual healing), physics (quantum approaches to consciousness and the holographic view of the mind) and ecology (deep ecology and the Gaia hypothesis of Earth as a conscious being). And in the nonprofessional mainstream of America, even the mass media have become involved with this new world view. In books (with recent bestsellers including *The Celestine Prophecy, Embraced by the Light, Conversations with God*, and *Caring for the Soul*), in movies (from "Ghost" and "Defending Your Life" to "Phenomenon" and "Contact"), on television ("The X-Files" and its clones), and in music (the whole genre of New Age music designed to induce specific changes in awareness), there is a burgeoning interest in what has loosely become known as New Age spirituality.

Despite the welter of apparently unrelated topics that often coalesce under this title, it is possible to discern some overriding patterns that can help us make sense of this jumbled spectrum of ideas. One metaphor I find particularly useful in understanding this array of phenomena involves comparing the human mind to a radio. Our brain receives thoughts, rather than creates them. Imagine further that we in the West have traditionally been taught that our mental radios can receive only one station, called normal waking consciousness (this station is also called the beta state by EEG researchers). More recently, a second frequency or station has been acknowledged as important by our scientists, the alpha state that enhances relaxation.

But most currently, various psycho-technologies are providing each human being with the means to tune in to an entire spectrum or frequency band of consciousness, not just the one or two stations we have become accustomed to. In the past 30 years, America's collective radio dials have been shaken loose from their fixed positions by the various chemical and herbal means discovered and rediscovered from the 1960s onward. Our current proliferation of holistic therapies and psychological schools promises to teach each person to use his mental radio to its fullest potential, tuning into information at the physical, psychological, emotional, conceptual, and spiritual levels.

One of the most important techniques for shifting one's radio tuner is a process of attentional focus which underlies so many of these New Age (and classical) spiritual techniques that it can even be called the final common denominator of altered states of consciousness. I am referring to the technique of hypnosis.

Hypnosis has long been misunderstood by the general public because of a Hollywood-instigated focus on its use as a form of involuntary mind control. But hypnosis is now taking its rightful place at the forefront of the new medical system known as mind/body medicine. Research has now validated many of the somewhat amazing claims of hypnotherapists, and the emerging field of psychoneuroimmunology (PNI) relies quite extensively on hypnosis to provide cues and suggestions to a patient's unconscious mind. National Institutes of Health studies are finally beginning to unravel the mind/body mechanisms which underly hypnosis.

Surprisingly, though, the field of clinical hypnosis has become staid in its own way, even though it is perceived by conventional medicine as an innovative and unconventional technique. By focusing on the mind/body aspects of PNI, mainstream hypnosis has lost touch with its transformative and transpersonal potential. Partially due to fear of losing its hard-earned mainstream credibility, organized hypnosis has not fully embraced the manifold spiritual applications of hypnosis. Yet my experiences in giving numerous lectures and workshops on transpersonal topics over the past nine years, coupled with an active hospital-based practice in mind/body medicine focused on pain management, have convinced me that there is an increasing interest in these formerly taboo or "off-the-wall" topics.

This more "mainstream" form of medical hypnosis represents only one small portion of what hypnosis enables a participant to experience. For these medical uses still involve the participant in his or her normal self-concept; entering a state of deep relaxation and using mental images to create suggestions for physical health does not require a new view of what it means to possess human awareness. It is a relief to find a classical FM station to supplement the Top 40's AM station that used to be the listener's mainstay, but there is still much more out there. The entire shortwave spectrum is still undiscovered by users of traditional medical hypnosis.

However, there is another cluster of hypnotherapeutic strategies which *does* demand a radical rethinking of what we are about. These are the techniques that bring us to an awareness of our transpersonal nature. That part of us that remains even after we have accounted for our physical body, our thoughts and emotions, our personalities and our memories — this is the transpersonal self, the spiritual realm, the shortwave band. Mysticism has long been the province of religious disciplines, but we now see psychologists and physicians becoming interested in spiritual topics such as out-of-body experiences, past life therapy, soul retrieval, clairvoyant diagnosis. These are the abilities and experiences that stem from our transpersonal nature, and they are the subject of this book. I have tried to bring together spokespersons for some of the most intriguing, if controversial, applications of transpersonal hypnotherapeutic techniques, to provide the reader with an overview of these sorts of transpersonal applications of hypnosis.

This spiritual dimension is not only an issue for clinicians as it pervades everyday life in fascinating ways. This omnipresence explains the current fascination. Even the process of editing this book illustrates the perplexing yet enticing nature of spiritual awareness, in a way that is worthy of mention.

The initial phase of organizing this book was marked by a burst of the sort of exuberant creative energy that gets authors hooked on their craft. The outline and several chapter drafts came together so effortlessly that I assumed this project was destined to succeed, until I then encountered a series of striking setbacks. My answering machine broke down and did not save key messages, the computer disk storing the book's contents got mysteriously reconfigured into an arcane and inaccessable format (apparently induced by the nearby office air ionizer that somehow spared all the other disks in the stack). I even spent some time in the hospital recovering from an unlikely infection that seemed to symbolize my frustrations. At that point I decided to practice what I was preaching and seek help from a friend who knew how to access information from the nether reaches of that metaphorical radio band.

In other words, I had a psychic consultation. In a modified self-hypnotic trance, a colleague of mine was able to "receive" information from her so-called spirit guides, via a process that is described more fully in Chapter 13 of this book. I was told that the book project had gotten bogged down because it had become tainted with my own "ego" energy; I was now perceiving the book as my personal creation and my ticket to fame. The initial burst of energy and progress was marked by a more selfless attitude, and so was readily supported by the universe as the project proceeded effortlessly. But the more my ego intervened, the more my work on the book project sputtered. Further, acccording to this psychic friend, the major purpose of the book had already been accomplished, even though it hadn't yet been published. I was told that my job had really been to accumulate ideas about transpersonal hypnosis and place these ideas on the information grid which encompasses the earth (much like the noosphere in de Chardin's *The Phenomenon of Man*), so that other people could access this information telepathically in the dream state.

My initial reaction to this information was to laugh in disbelief. It took me several months to digest this information, and to expand my belief system to encompass these possibilities. But then a new phase of the book's growth began when I started to acknowledge consciously that my collaborators and I were jointly performing a service to other students of consciousness. We were making important information more readily accessible to them, whether in the published hardcopy form that my ego preferred, or in the intangible realm of the alleged mental Internet that we all supposedly study from during our dream journeys. From that point on, things fell into place: the text was readily assembled and a recalcitrant publisher was replaced with a cooperative one.

This change in my own perspective, from ego-centered to (relatively) selfless, is a shift from what I am calling the personal to the transpersonal viewpoint. This shift is accompanied by a growing sense of equanimity, compassion, and purpose, and it is marked by a decrease in fear. This distinction between personal and transpersonal levels of being will be highlighted by the various techniques discussed in this book and will hopefully leave the reader with a greater appreciation for man's spiritual complexity and depth. Man's nature is seen as multidimensional, encompassing the entire range of radio frequencies, both personal and transpersonal.

This book is organized in such a way that the reader can at any point locate him or herself in the appropriate dimension within the transpersonal domain. Each chapter will follow a similar organization, beginning with an outline of the development of that particular technique or approach and highlighting where it falls in the history of hypnotherapy. Next, underlying theoretical principles are outlined, and then, in the heart of each chapter, several actual clinical vignettes will be presented to highlight the types of medical and psychological symptoms which are responsive to these approaches. Relevant references from the professional literature will be provided, with an emphasis on experimental studies which examine the validity of these techniques. Finally, each author will provide some resources to enable the interested reader to pursue further professional development in these areas, ranging from a list of appropriate training programs to a directory of skilled practioners nationwide.

The underlying model of human consciousness that pervades this book is the energy field model, or the spectrum of consciousness model. Each quality of human consciousness is seen to have a particular energetic frequency on this vibrational spectrum (analogous to the aforementioned radio dial), as well as a corresponding physical location in the subtle anatomy of the human energy field. This model will be explicated in more detail in the second chapter, and then each subsequent chapter's hypnotherapeutic technique will be shown to impact one particular level or aspect of the human energy field. In other words, each hypnotic technique allows the participant to tune his mental radio to one more new station.

To finish this introduction with another metaphor, I hope that this book will provide a rudimentary road map of the world of transpersonal hypnotherapies. Interested explorers can use this as a basic guide if they are just beginning their journeys, or as a way to reorient themselves at midjourney in their own professional and personal lives. Hopefully these transpersonal techniques and attitudes will help us reconnect with those deeper parts of ourselves that are most fully spiritual and therefore most fully human.

Chapter Summaries

Most of the topics addressed in this book are guaranteed to stir up controversy in traditional mental health circles. Part of this resistance stems from a denial of the reality of paranormal or psychic phenomena, whether simple hunches and intuitive flashes, or more dramatic remote viewing and pre-cognition. This widespread resistance to psi phenomena (psychic phenom-ena), both personal and institutional resistance, is important to appreciate, even before we plunge into the various hypnotic techniques described in this book. This book will start with remarks by a pioneer in the field of altered states of consciousness. In Chapter 1, Charles Tart summarizes his recent thoughts in a way which challenges us all to examine the limitations in our current belief systems. The extent to which emotion can color our scientific understanding becomes clear in this paper.

The next three chapters are bound by their focus on the model that will become the basic framework for this book, the human energy field. Begin-ning with the work of Franz Anton Mesmer, and evolving through clinical hypnosis into modern biomagnetism, the language of energy field dynamics will be introduced as a way to understand the various transpersonal tech-niques that will be described throughout this book. The history of hypnosis represents an important branching off point from the mainstream of scientific progress, during which these exotic notions were thoroughly explored.

In Chapter 2, I look at the work of the notorious Franz Anton Mesmer; his prescient foray into Animal Magnetism will be re-examined in light of modern discoveries in the field of biomagnetism. "Mesmerism" will be shown to have important differences and similarities to clinical hypnosis, even though the terms are often loosely used as synonyms. This work sug-gests that biomagnetic fields can be manipulated directly (through Mesmeric passes of the hands), or indirectly (through hypnotic words and images).

Chapter 3 extends this notion of healing with the human energy field by considering the ancient art of the laying on of hands as a trance phenom-enon. In this section, I explore in more detail the physical configuration of the energy field, man's so-called subtle anatomy.

The pathways for the circulation of life energy, and the central collecting points for its storage and transmission will be shown to underlie healing techniques ranging from acupuncture to massage. Different levels, or sheaths, of the energy body will provide a road map for understanding where each of the different hypnotic techniques in this book has its most direct impact.

In Chapter 4, John Tatum expands on the model of energy fields to demonstrate how energetic resonance between two neighboring fields can explain important subjective events in clinical practice. He describes how intuition, empathy, hunches, and flashes of insight, may be an effect of sympathetic resonance, the collaborative trance that occurs between the therapist and the patient. Learning to tune in to subtle sensations from our own energy centers can make us all the more intuitive and empathic thera-pists, and can certainly lead to a heightened appreciation for the many subtle ways that people interact, interpersonally and transpersonally, when in a hypnotherapeutic setting.

Chapters 5 through 8 all reflect transpersonal psychology's debt to the spiritual practice of yoga, from breathwork to body postures to energy centers to meditation. In Chapter 5, Susana Galle integrates yogic bodywork with trance practices to elicit deep healing in a number of clinical situations. She demonstrates an effective integration of East and West in her work, and illustrates how the different languages of two superficially different transpersonal traditions can be effectively synthesized.

In Chapter 6, Darlene Osowiec focuses on a specific yogic technique for regulating the flow of life energy, the conscious control of the pattern of breathing. She describes how recent work with ultradian rhythms and trance cycles is connected to this ancient yogic practice. She describes research which interrelates ultradian biologic rhythms with hypnotic susceptibility and with various patterns of breath flow.

In Chapter 7, Stephen Gallegos outlines his synthesis of guided imagery with the energy center model of yoga. He helps clients contact inner guidance in the form of totem animal images that represent the emotional functions of each yogic energy center. Though he does not use the language of formal hypnosis to describe his work, his blending of shamanic journeying and Eastern subtle anatomy leads to profound psychological reintegration.

In Chapter 8, Steven Wolinsky compares and contrasts meditation with hypnosis in their effects on consciousness. He sees meditation as a way of "de-hypnotizing" patients from their symptom-producing trances of everyday life. Meditation helps people to develop the witness position of pure awareness. By no longer identifying with the contents of the personality, we can begin to identify with the transpersonal parts of our being.

The final five chapters of this book look at the bridge between the individual personality or ego state, and the higher self or soul. They consider the individual energy body as a springboard to the transpersonal self. In Chapter 9, Roger Woolger moves his clients beyond an identification with the story of their current life by helping them access memories of past lives. He believes that these stories can be taken as helpful metaphors that facilitate healing, or as forgotten stories of the soul's passages through other lifetimes. Using the Jungian perspective of archetypal knowledge, Woolger describes one case example in detail. By understanding the lessons of each lifetime, we gain an appreciation of the soul's true nature.

If the soul can travel through various life stories, then it must exist *in toto* even between lives; and if there is a life after death, then there must also be a life before birth. David Chamberlain has worked for over 30 years in accessing memories of deep awareness during intra-uterine life, supposedly before the nervous system has matured enough to register memories (at least according to orthodox science). His specific clinical examples in Chapter 10 suggest that there is a transpersonal part of our awareness that is continuous before birth and after death.

Joseph Wicker addresses the problem of those personality entities who do not make a graceful passage out of their earthly focus when they die. Out of confusion and fear, some choose to remain involved in human affairs becoming so entwined with other living people that they need to be extricated in a process called spirit releasement.

Related to exorcism, this hypnotic process has led to striking therapeutic changes in appropriately chosen patients. Mindful of potential religious controversy, Wicker draws on his extensive theological training to tread this territory carefully and respectfully in Chapter 11.

Many nonwestern cultures are quite comfortable with these transpersonal domains and integrate them into their healing practices. In Chapter 12, Stanley Krippner gives a transcultural view of the processes of spirit healing and mediumship to highlight the universal nature of these experiences. He focuses in detail on two indigenous traditions which exemplify the use of what might be called the transcultural transpersonal trance.

The Western approach to communicating with spirits has its roots in Biblical prophecy and is enjoying a resurgence today in its current incarnation as channeling. In my survey of this phenomenon in Chapter 13, I do not focus on the problematic question of its alleged factual validity. Instead I review some of the experimental psychology literature in this area, and then I provide readers with samples of what I consider to be high quality information that has become available to us through the medium of trance mediums. Further references are also provided, for more detailed channeled information on health issues, physics and cosmology, personal psychology, American politics, and Earth's role in the evolution of our universe. Perhaps the medium is the message, after all.

With these brief descriptions to provide your roadmap in hand, I wish you well on your transpersonal journey.

Acknowledgments

I thank my fellow contributors, without whose help there would be no book, and the American Society of Clinical Hypnosis, whose conferences provided the forum for meeting so many of these colleagues. I am grateful to Spaulding Rehabilitation Hospital's Pain Management Program (inpatient and outpatient), where my colleagues still make it fun to go to work. I thank the Monday night healer's group for providing a supportive sounding board, and the Williamstown community (especially the Men's Lodge) for starting me on this road many years ago.

I'd like to honor the memory of the three teachers who most inspired my work: Henry Fortier, Dr. Earl Ettienne, and most importantly Dr. Sidney Leskowitz, my father. I also thank those unnamed friends, colleagues, and patients whose search for wholeness continues to inspire me.

And finally, I am grateful for the loving support of my family, both the extended branches and the nuclear one: Shari, David, and especially Doreen. Now I know how hard it is for a few words of acknowledgment to capture the essence of the love and support that make things happen.

Eric Leskowitz, M.D.

Contributors

David Chamberlain, Ph.D. is a psychologist practicing in San Diego, CA. He served as President of the Association for Pre- and Peri-natal Psychology and Health (APPPAH) for eight years and is founding editor of birthpsychology.com on the World Wide Web. With over 40 published works, he is a major contributor to pre- and perinatal psychology. His book *The Mind of Your Newborn Baby*, 3rd Ed., (1998) is available in eight languages. Email: wombpsi@msn.com.

Susana A. Hassan-Schwarz Galle, Ph.D. is the founder and director of the Body/Mind Center in Washington D.C., where she practices holistic psychotherapy. She studied at UC Berkeley and Yale, and is an Assistant Clinical Professor of Pediatrics at Georgetown Medical School, and Allied Doctoral Scientist in Adolescent Medicine at George Washington Medical School. She is certified as a yoga therapist and teacher, and is on the editorial board of *The Journal of Pre- and Peri-Natal Psychology*.

Eligio Stephen Gallegos, Ph.D., holds degress from the University of Wisconsion, New Mexico State University, and Florida State University. He is former chairman of the Psychology Department at Mercer University, and Honorary Director of the International Institute for Visualization Research. He offers workshops and trains people around the world in the use of imagery in communication and psychotherapy. He has contributed articles to professional journals and has written four books, including *Into Wholeness*, to be published in 1998.

Stanley Krippner, Ph.D., is a Professor of psychology at Saybrook Institute Graduate School in San Francisco. He is co-author of *The Mythic Path, Spiritual Dimensions of Healing,* and *Dream Telepathy,* and editor of *Dreamtime and Dreamwork* and *Broken Images, Broken Selves: Dissociative Narratives in Clinical Practice.* He has been president of the Association for Humanistic Psychology, the Association for the Study of Dreams, the Parapsychological Association, and three divisions of the American Psychological Association. Email: Skrippner@igc.apc.org.

Eric D. Leskowitz, M.D. is a Board Certified Psychiatrist who works with the Pain Management Program at Spaulding Rehabilitation Hospital in Boston. He holds clinical appointments to the departments of Psychiatry at Tufts and Harvard Medical Schools. He has studied energy healing for 10 years and has led seminars on energy medicine and consciousness for medical professionals both nationally and internationally. His articles have appeared in *Advances, Psychiatric Times, Natural Health, Subtle Energies,* and *Alternative Therapies in Health and Medicine.* Email: Rleskowitz@pol.net.

Darlene A. Osowiec, Ph.D. earned her Ph.D. in Clinical Psychology from the California Institute of Integral Studies, and an M.A. in Clinical Psychology from Roosevelt University, Chicago; she has done postgraduate work at the Saybrook Institute. She has been a student of meditation since 1970. In her Chicago-based private practice, Maximum Potential, she integrates Existential, Humanistic and Transpersonal perspectives into her work. Dr. Osowiec is currently serving as the Education and Training Chair of the American Psychological Association (APA) Division 30, Psychological Hypnosis. She's listed in "Who's Who in America" and "Who's Who in the World."

Charles T. Tart, Ph.D. is Visiting Professor at the California Institute of Integral Studies, and is a Professor Emeritus in the Department of Psychology at the University of California, Davis. He has authored or edited 13 books (including the classic *Altered States of Consciousness*) and over 200 articles, is on the editorial board of 12 journals, and is a member of 15 professional societies. He is currently president of the Parapsychological Association, and vice president elect of the Association of Humanistic Psychology. Email: Cttart@ucdavis.edu.

John Tatum, M.D. is a psychiatrist who trained at the Sheppard and Enoch Pratt Hospital and who specializes in psychotherapy and personal growth. He has had extensive training in subtle energies with Brugh Joy, and with the Nine Gates Mystery School as participant and assistant. He is a Second Degree Reiki practitioner, and a Second Degree Black Belt and teacher in Aikido. He has used energetic intuition and interaction in his psychotherapy practice for 13 years. Email: Jtatum@magicnet.net.

Joseph Wicker, Psy.D. has studied Transpersonal Psychology since 1970, and has been practicing hypnosis since 1983. He has an M.A. in philosphy from the Athenaeum of Ohio, an M.A. in theology from the University of Dayton, and he did doctoral studies in theology at Fordham University. His Psy.D. in psychology is from Wright State University. Dr. Wicker has been in private practice in Cincinnati, OH since 1984 with the Behavioral Science Center.

Stephen Wolinsky, Ph.D. began his clinical practice in Los Angeles in 1974 as a Gestalt and Reichian therapist. In 1977 he journeyed to India, where he lived for 6 years studying meditation. His integration of these fields with Ericksonian Hypnosis and NLP has led to the publication of three books in addition to *Trances People Live: Healing Approaches in Quantum Psychology* (1991). He offers year-long trainings in hypnosis, psychotherapy, and family therapy, and is director of the Quantum Psychology Institute in New Mexico.

Roger J. Woolger, Ph.D. is a British born Jungian analyst, past-life therapist, and lecturer on cultural psychology. He holds degrees from Oxford and London Universities, and the C. G. Jung Insitutute in Zurich, and has taught at Vassar College, University of Vermont, and Concordia University. His book *Other Lives, Other Selves* is a synthesis of his training in depth psychotherapy and bodywork, and has been translated into five languages. He gives workshops and seminars nationally and worldwide.

Contents

chapter one

Fear of psychic phenomena*

Charles T. Tart

Fear of the paranormal is not only a complex topic, it is also not an easy topic to discuss for a natural optimist such as myself, whose preferred way of dealing with fears is to forget about them and hope that they never materialize. Fear is not simply an intellectual topic; it is an intensely emotional topic. I am interested in understanding consciousness, and I have proposed the idea of "state-specific sciences:" to *really* observe and fully understand particular phenomena, such as fear, you have to be in a fear-dominated state of consciousness.

This chapter will discuss fear of the paranormal, of the transpersonal, and of the kind of "subtle energies" phenomena so many therapists are now working with. I do not have final answers, so my basic goal is to stir up readers. It is a topic that really has to be thought about, though, and it has to be dealt with in various ways. Fear is something that runs around in the background all the time and distorts what we do in terms of trying to understand consciousness. Also, it distorts any attempts to apply our findings. And certainly it has a lot to do with whether this field of transpersonal research gets any acceptance from the scientific mainstream.

Many who work within a scientific setting, or have scientific or medical colleagues, say that science is the backbone of their practice. Usually when they say "science" they mean a combination of being logical, open minded, and curious, and letting the facts fall where they may. Those are the ideals of science. Science in its ideal form is actually a tremendous spiritual vocation with a commitment to stay open to reality no matter what one would like it to be. Certainly, scientists and physicians in general are quite proud of their objectivity and open-mindedness.

* This chapter was adapted from a keynote speech entitled "Fears of the Paranormal in ourselves and our Colleagues: Recognizing them, dealing with them," at the Annual Meeting of ISSSEEM, 1994.

Many researchers have done research and applications on topics such as subtle energies, and when they presented these results to colleagues they have not gotten very enthusiastic receptions (to put it mildly). Indeed they have found that criticisms seem to be more intense than the subject warranted. When I asked about this at a recent presentation of mine at the International Society for the Study of Subtle Energy and Energy Medicine (ISSSEEM), almost all attendees felt that they had been emotionally attacked, personally attacked, for their interests in the paranormal during the course of their careers, and have felt defensive. (Just because you know you're paranoid doesn't mean they aren't out to get you.)

Organizations such as ISSSEEM focus on energy medicine and subtle energies. Those are good scientific-sounding terms, undoubtedly chosen with the goal of inching a little bit further toward respectability. But that group mainly focuses on parapsychology. Whatever name is used, "parabiology," "paramedicine," etc., this subject is not part of the mainstream.

The prefix "para," as it is usually applied in parapsychology, means "beyond" or "alongside of." "Para" also means "incorrect" and "abnormal" in many applications. I have discovered that others often like that usage best with respect to what parapsychologists do.

Practicing paramedicine or parabiology or transpersonal psychology means to work contrary to the dominant materialistic paradigm. In fact, this work is antimaterialistic, or more accurately, anti-*scientistic*. Not anti-scientific, because there is no conflict between what we do and genuine science, genuine open-mindedness to reality. But current findings in science and related fields of discourse have tended to become fossilized and defended as in a fundamentalist religion (scientism) with its own Inquisition, so what we are doing is definitely anti-scientistic.

In this chapter, I will share briefly what I have learned in parapsychological research over the last 30 years about the kinds of fears and resistances that usually work in the background and affect what we do and learn, in the hope that the field of transpersonal therapies might learn something from these fears and resistances and not go through the suffering that formal parapsychology has gone through.

Technically, we do not really know what we are doing when we talk about energy medicine. Nevertheless, there is something there, and it is something important. We have theories sometimes, but we do not really know, in any very satisfactory way, the details. Nevertheless, we need to learn about these subtle energy and parapsychological phenomena, simply for aid in understanding what is the nature of existence.

As an example of the kind of resistance that occurs on an overt level to parapsychological findings, consider the work of the late Charles Honorton, one of the great parapsychologists. He kept an extensive file over the course of many years and found that various parapsychologists submitted studies to *Science*; their articles were all rejected. Charles Honorton studied the reasons that were given for rejection and found that if the submission was a paper that presented empirical data showing some parapsychological effect, the usual reason given for rejection stated that since there was no proper theoretical understanding of this, there was no point in publishing it because the data didn't make sense. On the other hand, if the paper was theoretical, it was rejected on the grounds that there were no empirical data to support this kind of theorizing. It is a sad and revealing story that illustrates the illogical, irrational resistance side of the scientific establishment. I strongly believe in the ideals of science. But science is performed by real people who have normal human "hang ups" and have real problems when they come face to face with the paranormal and the transpersonal.

Another example of the degree of resistance this field generates is that there is a very active international organization devoted to debunking it. Sometimes detractors talk about the money being wasted on parapsychology research, but, in fact, the money spent on parapsychology research is *trivial*. I did a survey years ago and found that *all* the laboratories in the United States and Canada put together spent only half a million dollars a year, which might otherwise buy a half minute commercial on national television.[1] So it is not the waste of money that is the real issue.

It is easy to understand how some people get incensed about charlatans who claim they are doing something psychic or spiritual, and are clearly fraudulent. But why would they go out of their way to stop scientific research, especially if these organizations were really skeptical and scientific? "Skeptic" means not having made up your mind but looking at the evidence. I believe it would be more helpful if they were helping us get grant money instead of opposing our research attempts. It does not make sense to me.

Admittedly there has always been a rational component to this resistance to parapsychological research, and that has led to the injunction to conduct higher quality experiments. The result has been that the methodological quality of experiments in formal parapsychology, by and large, is much better than in any other area of science. There has been so much criticism of parapsychology for so long that the methodology has become very stringent and there is no rational way to dismiss rigorous evidence.

Such a high level of methodological rigor is not the case yet in energy medicine. From this rational perspective, experimental designs should be made as rigorous as possible. Casual experiments are not for publication. If a researcher wants more than casual conversation about "something interesting I've seen," a researcher must be rigorous. Sloppily designed experiments, when published, will be criticized and treated as if they are typical of the field. Debunkers almost never refer to studies that are methodologically of high quality.

Methodological standards have to be high. New experimentalists, even those who really understand subtle energy, can learn the methodology by reading the *Handbook of Parapsychology* by Benjamin Wolman and colleagues.[2] Enroll in the course at the Rhine Institute for Parapsychology offered in Durham, N.C. each summer to learn basic methodology.

The subject of hypnosis raises many of these issues. Back in the early and middle 1960s, I specialized in hypnosis research. I was truly impressed by the power of hypnosis, and I still am. Though I have done a substantial amount of work in the field, I could never get over the fact that I could sit down and talk to a client for fifteen or twenty minutes, and, for some people, their total reality changed. I've never understood, therefore, why hypnosis is a fringe topic in psychology. The effects are a thousand times bigger than almost all things psychologists study.

I was interested in all aspects of hypnosis and that included reading much of the older literature in which psychic abilities seemed to routinely become available in deep hypnotic states abilities such as telepathic hypnosis. I was fascinated by these very powerful experiences, I wanted to do similar studies, and yet I also felt ambivalent. Did I really want psychic abilities to manifest strongly? In many of my workshops, I've found that people would rather not have psychic power, and I will outline the most common reasons for this.[4,5]

In an initial formal inquiry as to why people would have negative feelings about psychic abilities, based on my years of informal study, I and Katie LaBore individually asked people to seriously imagine that they could take a treatment that would allow them a permanent, telepathically read/know the thoughts and feelings of everyone who was physically near them. Reactions to imagining acquiring this ability were predominantly negative. Common concerns expressed included worries about controlling the ability, incapacitating overload, the responsibility such a capacity created towards others, their lack of maturity to deal with such responsibility, and fears of rejection by others if they learned of this telepathic ability. Some even worried about confusing the thoughts and feelings of others with their own. We don't expect psychic abilities to work this well in the laboratory, but how much of this kind of ambivalence exists when subjects are asked to use psychic abilities in laboratory experiments?

Let's switch now to talking about researchers, experimenters in parapsychology, rather than the subjects.

In parapsychology, unfortunately, there is a long running myth, taken over straight from psychology, about the objective experimenter who works with subjects. There is an assumption that the researcher is superior to the subjects. The experimenter *subjects* people to things. This can distort results in psychology in general, and this happens in parapsychology, also. Because of this belief in objectivity, researchers supposedly do not have any problem with irrational things such as fears of psi.

Unfortunately, that is not really the case, as I will demonstrate by discussing telepathic hypnosis. Dr. Jule Eisenbud was a psychoanalyst who contributed a great deal to our understanding of this field. He made a list of successful experiments in parapsychology over the last 75 years that, after tremendous initial success, have not been performed again,[6] specifically the telepathic hypnosis trials done at the end of the last century by Pierre Janet and other people.

In a series of experiments which Janet reported some months after his early work, Leone, his highly trained telepathic subject, was not only repeatedly hypnotized at a distance in the presence of several lay and medical witnesses, but was also made to carry out posthypnotic commands given mentally. Of 21 trials done over a period of days, at distances of at least 500 meters, no less than 16 were judged a compete success. The times for the trials were randomly chosen. All trials in which Leone was not found in deep trance when the investigators entered her house, or when the trance did not follow the mental suggestion within a quarter of an hour, were counted as failures. During this entire period, Leone fell into only two trances which were considered spontaneous and outside the experimental program. Another time when she had been incompletely awakened from a previous cataleptic state and had done nothing but doze in the intervening two hours, the posthypnotic commands which were successfully carried out were simple acts, such as going into another room and lighting the lamp in broad daylight.

In other words, they were not the sort of things that would happen spontaneously. Evaluating these results, Janet wrote, "Are we to imagine that on 16 occasions there was a rather exact coincidence? Such a supposition is a little unreasonable. Was there at any time involuntary suggestion on our part? All I can say, and I say this with utmost sincerity, is that we took every possible precaution to avoid this." Eisenbud further states that the now celebrated Leone was subsequently studied by Charles Richet, professor of physiology at the faculty of medicine of the University of Paris, and later a Nobel Prize winner. Richet successfully duplicated the results of Janet and Gilbert. Besides those of Janet, four other papers on telepathic hypnosis were read before the Society of Physiological Psychology in the winter of 1885 and the spring of 1886.

But, Eisenbud states, now comes the puzzling thing. With the exception of one well-written account of hypnosis experiments on traveling clairvoyance by a Swedish physician in 1892, practically all work on the telepathic aspects of hypnosis came to a standstill by the end of the decade in which its most significant and most promising results were achieved. One could imagine that the writers of these reports might have felt something of the surprise of Cortez catching his first breathtaking view of the Pacific. Those who wrote of these experiments might have sensed that no other studies they were likely to pursue could possibly match in importance the experiments they had barely embarked upon. They would have starved, if need be, to continue such investigations that might have held the key to profound enigmas in biology, medicine, anthropology, sociology, and philosophy. But nothing like this developed. Janet suddenly found that the quirks of his hysterical patients at the Salpetriere presented a much more rewarding field of study, and Richet returned to his physiology and other types of psychic phenomena. Of the others, history does not tell.

In 1925, most standard texts on hypnotism no longer mentioned the telepathic aspects at all. Janet himself wrote, "Such a decadence, so rapid a disappearance after such high enthusiasm and such extensive developments is certainly surprising." He confessed that he could no longer quite understand how he got the results he had reported in 1886. Although he did not flatly disavow what he had reported in good faith at the time, it is clear that he had great difficulty believing that such things had happened. It was like a dim and distant dream, or a childhood memory which was no longer trustworthy. It is very interesting that an eminent researcher would abandon such clearcut findings.

Parapsychologists are an unusual group. For more than 20 years I attended conventions of the Parapsychological Association, which is the scientific body in this field. Over the years I noticed a very interesting phenomenon that I named "The Religion of the .05 Level" that I will discuss in more detail later in this chapter. If a parapsychologist presented an experimental study that involved some kind of repeated guessing, and the results were reported to be statistically significant (i.e., you would know that they would occur by chance alone less than five times out of a hundred) there might be some criticisms of the methodology, but generally not, because reports were reviewed by the Parapsychological Association's program committee first.

But statistical significance can be achieved while the amount of psi demonstrated is trivial. Guessing red or black on a deck of cards will average 50% by chance alone, and if someone averages 50.5% over a long period of time, that can be very *statistically* significant, but it means they are guessing 99.5% of the time. It is only once in a great while that anything psychic happens. That is intellectually stimulating for parapsychologists, but it does not really bring much psi home or make it real to the average person.

On the other hand, when a researcher would occasionally present a paper concerning extensive amounts of ESP manifesting, the amount and intensity of methodological criticism would be astounding. In fact, parapsychologists are the severest critics of other parapsychologists who get strong psychic results in the laboratory.[7]

I have several theories to explain why people might not use psychic abilities, or why they might be afraid of them. In an article I wrote for the *Journal of Parapsychology,* I named the first theory a social-masking theory of psychic inhibition. Part of being a normal social person means having an implicit contract with others. For example, "I would like to be known to you on *my* terms, and if you will honor them, you can be known to me on *your* terms." That's not perfect of course, because we see many things about others they'd prefer us not to see, and we also expose things about ourselves we don't want to.

The implicit social contract calls for not knowing each other very well; we uphold our own self-image to avoid facing things we don't want to know about ourselves. Having other people uphold our illusions helps us uphold our own defenses. (Besides, how would you sell your used car if we had really strongly functioning psi in general?)

There are many social pressures that we do not even see. They were built into us so long ago that we do not think about certain kinds of things or do certain things. I'm not saying people get up in the morning and need to remind themselves, "I will not be psychic today. I will behave." It happens automatically. (It might be an interesting experiential exercise, though, to say that to yourself a few mornings in a row, keeping it in mind and seeing what happens.)

In addition to the social masking theory there is a deeper level of psychological theorizing that I call the *primal conflict* theory of psi inhibition. I believe it is likely that infants and mothers have a great deal of telepathic communication starting sometime while the baby is still in the womb. It is not verbal communication, but a feeling communication. My belief is this is perfectly natural, and it is a psychic bond that persists for some time after birth, perhaps up to a period of years. David Chamberlain's work on perinatal hypnosis (see Chapter 10) explores this bond in great detail later in this book.

In my primal conflict theory, I believe we grow up in a society that has rules about how we are supposed to perceive the world, what we are supposed to believe about it, how we are supposed to think, how we are supposed to feel, how we are supposed to behave. Consequently I believe this primal telepathic link causes problems between mothers and young children. For example, it is difficult for a mother to hide her displeasure with a child, especially when the child has gotten into trouble, broken an object, or made a mess. A mother will often try to explain patiently to the child about the error, but the feelings of anger within the mother are often perceived by the child due to this primal link.

Children receive this double message verbally on the conscious level, of social acceptability and telepathically on the unconscious level, this primal, emotional level.

In an attempt to cope with this conflict, perhaps there is a general repression of psychic abilities, to shut off that channel so the intense emotions do not come through consciously, and then the conflict "disappears." However, this is not ultimately healthy: repression per se is not a healthy defense mechanism because you cut out part of reality. But I believe that primal conflict repression accounts for a general lack of psychic functioning in society, and it also may explain some of the intense levels of resistance to the appearance of psychic abilities. For example, a critic may argue heatedly about the trivial points of methodological design in some psi experiments. Maybe at some level the unconscious mind says, "To look seriously at telepathy is to remember mother's rejection, and that's totally unacceptable." The unconscious can easily put things like this together.

One more theory that I have relevant to fear of psi, I will call the repression of our spiritual self. From my point of view, we are basically spiritual beings, and we are here in this interesting planetary spiritual school. But the particular classroom we're in discounts spirituality in favor of scientific materialism. To deny a spiritual self is a way to avoid having to consciously live with the conflicts of disappointment, and cultural disapproval for being "spiritual."

I believe militant denial of the spiritual is a result of this repression. There's a lot of psychological pressure underneath. And, even worse, suppose that spiritual stuff is true? One may say, "I'm supposed to make something spiritual of my life, and I've just been having fun, getting ahead and making money. There's nothing to that spiritual stuff anyway, so I've got nothing to worry about." The idea of opening to the psychic stuff, which maybe starts opening to the spiritual, threatens to raise these kinds of conflicts. So repression of our "higher selves," our transpersonal selves, may be a very real factor here.

I would now like to discuss eleven psychological methods for dealing with the fears of psychic material (also see Reference 9). Five of these methods are not completely satisfactory because they have a pathological element, or there's some kind of high psychological cost. The other six are healthier. The first of the five methods (a very popular one) of dealing with fear of psi is to simply deny that psi exists: "It does not exist, therefore, I am not afraid of it." A slight variant of that is to accept psi but deny that you're afraid of it even though you actually are.

A second very common method for dealing with fear of psi is avoidance, staying away from situations that might trigger it. Some people are very good at it. For instance, the many scientists who are prominent pseudo-skeptics can claim quite genuinely they have never seen any evidence that convinces them of the existence of psi for they have never looked at it.

Another way of avoiding circumstances that trigger fear of psi is a technique used by many parapsychologists, and it is to zealously practice "The Religion of the .05 Level." Some researchers design experiments in such a way that *intellectually,* through statistical analysis, results indicate some psi happened, but it is of such a low magnitude that it does not make a significant impression on the researcher. I performed some studies in which people were using a 10-choice trainer, where they had 10 possibilities on each try. You don't get many hits by chance on that. The average is one out of ten, and if anyone could average one-and-a-half or two, they were outstanding. One person who started in this training procedure, improved until she was averaging four and five. She then broke into tears and quit the study. Psi was too real. I believe it crossed the "gut-level" reality threshold and triggered her psi-fear problem, which wasn't resolved.

Another common way of dealing with fear is by rationalization. For instance, a person might say, "No, no, all this psychic stuff comes from the higher realms of the spirit and is only good." Now that might be true. But it's an evasion and rationalization. It's easier to sweep any frightening aspects of psi under the table. All of these evasions have a high price.

There is the distraction method of dealing with fear of psi. Some parapsychologists become so obsessed with the technical details of their experiments and methodologies, they never notice that something is actually happening. It is a common professional habit. One becomes a better and better methodologist but never actually finishes any experiments because of fine tuning the procedure.

Then there is the dissociation way of defense against fear of psi. "I don't do it, I just channel the spirits. I'm not psychic, it's in the cards, it's in the tea leaves, it's in the horoscope, it's in the readings of the aura meter." This is a manifestation of what Kenneth Batcheldor, the late parapsychologist, called ownership resistance.[10] A medium or psychic person may act as if they did not have anything to do with it. They falsely project into the system, "It's not me, it's this psychic machine." Some systems may have an independent psi function, though I've never seen evidence of it, but it's quite clear that systems sometimes give people permission to use their own psychic abilities.

All of these methods I've mentioned so far are unhealthy in the sense that they deny certain aspects of reality. Let's talk about healthier defense mechanisms. The first method is what we might call the desensitization way of dealing with psi. Familiarizing oneself with the topic will help reduce a fear of it. This is something we do in many aspects of life. Something frightens us, but we keep doing it because we have to, and after a while we do not notice the fear. We become desensitized. In certain respects that is quite healthy. Sometimes, though, it can be a way of covering over the real problem, and just getting used to something to avoid having to admit that there is a problem.

Another way of dealing with fear is through the use of what I call bypass defenses. Some of Kenneth Batcheldor's research was excellent on this.[10] For example, he got people involved in old-fashioned, Victorian table-tipping situations in a dark room, with everyone around the table. The table was instrumented so that it might detect genuine psi effects. But since a group was involved, a person could say, "It wasn't me, it was the other people, who probably cheated. You know, maybe it was psi, or maybe the other people pushed on the table." People spread the blame out and don't have to deal with it.

The really healthy methods of dealing with fear deal with cognitive and affective acknowledgment. I emphasize that this has to be emotional, affective, not just cognitive. The admission process actually helps one cope with some fears of psi in and of itself. Many fears operate in a grossly exaggerated fashion simply because we won't admit that they are a fear, but once they are brought into the light of consciousness, they change.

That, though, doesn't handle all of the fears of psychic phenomena. Some have to be looked at in a much more specific fashion. But that first step of cognitively and affectively acknowledging fear, and then doing that same thing with other people, essentially joining the human race and admitting to other people you have some fears, is very effective. You must use discretion, but that method can help many people. And as the pressure decreases, one can look more specifically at what the fears are. Sometimes the insights alone enable one to then cope with them.

The next method of handling fear is learning adaptive coping skills. After acknowledging a fear, play with it. Try doing different things to see if it gets worse or better. Does it give you insight into it, or does it cause panic in such a way that you can't see what you're doing? Admit that it bothers you. It may seem dangerous from your perspective, but play with it. If you have an attitude toward psi that it is dangerous in some respect, you can stay aware of that attitude and experiment with strategies of nevertheless working with it in some way that minimizes the danger without being unrealistically careless.

We must also accept responsibility for the power aspects of psi. But in much of the world down through the ages people wanted to learn psychic abilities in order to have power over other people. That possibility does seem to exist. If you accept the fact that you could develop your psi and hurt others, I hope you realize those feelings in yourself by knowing them, and you will not be carried away by them.

And finally, the ultimate way of dealing with fear of psychic abilities is personal and spiritual growth. Anything and everything you do that helps you know yourself better, that integrates you more fully, that makes you less rigid and more open, makes you more compassionate, and puts you in more of a spiritual relationship to the transpersonal aspects of the universe, will at least in an indirect way, deal with the fear of psi (See References 11 and 12).

To conclude: I've opened up a can of worms in some ways by bringing up this material about fear, but it needs to be opened. Unconscious fears can control people, influence and distort actions and perceptions in unrealized ways.

In this paper I've emphasized the negative, even though I'm not a negative person. The larger context for me is that we're here in this body, but we are also something spiritual. I hesitate to put names on it, but we are here, and there is plenty of adventure and pleasure here, and lots of suffering also. Mainly there is a tremendous opportunity to learn. If we work it right, we can grow in compassion and wisdom. I like the analogy of this world as a spiritual training school. Life is a training course like the Marine Corps. It's a tough course, but if you pass it, you really learn how to focus yourself.[11,12]

I am very optimistic about life and psi. I do not have any final answers on fear, but I hope you have had some insights. If you continue to look inside when psi situations get that odd feeling to them, I'll be very pleased. And I think the field will move on.

References

1. Tart, C., A survey on negative uses, government interest and funding of psi, *Psi News*, 1, 2 1978, 3.
2. B. Wolman, L. Dale, G. Schmeidler, and M. Ullman, *Handbook of Parapsychology*, Van Nostrand Reinhold, New York, 1977.
3. Tart, C., Card Guessing Tests: learning paradigm of extinction paradigm, *J. Amer. Soc. Psychical Res.*, 60, 1966, 46–55.
4. Tart, C. and K. LaBore, Attitudes Toward Strongly Functioning Psi: a preliminary study, *J. Amer. Soc. Psychical Res.*, 80, 1986, 163–173.
5. Tart, C., Psychics' fear of psychic powers, *J. Amer. Soc. Psychical Res.*, 80, 1986, 279–292.
6. Eisenbud, J., *Psi and Psychoanalysis: Studies in Psychoanalysis of Psi Conditioned Behavior*, Grune & Stratton, New York, 1970.

7. Tart, C., *Learning to Use Extrasensory Perception*, University of Chicago Press, Chicago, IL, 1976.

8. Tart, C., The Controversy about Psi: two psychological theories, *J. Parapsychol.*, 446, 1982, 313–320.

9. Tart, C., Acknowledging and dealing with the fear of psi, *J. Amer. Soc. Psychical Res.*, 78, 1984, 133–143.

10. Batcheldor, K., Contributions to the theory of PK Induction from Sittergroup work, *J. Amer. Soc. Psychical Res.*, 78, 1984, 105–122.

11. Tart, C., *Waking Up: Overcoming the obstacles to human potential*, New Science Library, Boston, 1986.

12. Tart, C., *Living the Mindful Life*, Shambhala, Boston, 1994.

Correspondence:

Charles T. Tart, Ph.D.
Psychology Department
University of California at Davis
Davis, CA 95616
cttart@ucdavis.edu

Institute for Parasychology
Rhine Research Center
402 N. Buchanan Blvd.
Durham, NC 27701-1728
(919) 688-8241
www.rhine.org

Parapsychology Association
www.parapsych.org

chapter two

Mesmerism, hypnosis, and the human energy field

Eric D. Leskowitz

Introduction

Transpersonal applications of hypnosis are not new. Prior to the resurgence of interest in altered states of consciousness over the last 30 years via the human potential movement, there was one strand of the orthodox Western medical tradition which generated some surprisingly prescient discoveries about the multidimensional nature of human awareness. Though dismissed as quackery by the dominant medical institutions of the day, these teachings are now worth re-examining in the light of recent scientific advances. I am referring to the work two hundred years ago of Franz Anton Mesmer, the father of Animal Magnetism. By taking another look at his controversial theories and practices, we can gain an overview of the field of transpersonal hypnosis because his work highlights the distinction between hypnosis as a verbal transaction and hypnosis as a modifier of the human energy field. His work also suggests that energy field dynamics may actually underlie *all* healing processes.

Mesmer's work leads to two vital insights into the nature of human consciousness, both of which will be recurring themes throughout this book. On the one hand is the well-known but often ridiculed concept of animal magnetism, the supposed 'fluidium' which interconnects all living organisms in the universe. Recent discoveries in the field of biomagnetism point to some dramatic correspondences with Mesmer's major tenets and lead to the possibility that human beings do not end at their skin, but extend in all directions as an electromagnetic field. Science is ready to prove that humans have a layer of subtle anatomic organization similiar to that described by such Eastern occult traditions as yoga and acupuncture. There is now a scientific basis for considering such phenomena as the aura or human energy field and such healing practices as the laying on of hands. This notion of a hierarchy of subtle energy structures that can be directly worked with in the trance state is one of the core insights of transpersonal schools of psychology, and so will be discussed at some length in the book (especially in Chapter 3 on energy healing, Chaper 4 on intuition, and Chapter 7 on the Personal Totem Pole Process).

The second Mesmeric insight, drawn more from the work of several of Mesmer's students than from the master himself, involves the discovery of a facet of individual consciousness that is clearly transpersonal. In fact, a school of his French disciples seems to have found a method of directly contacting the higher self, or the soul, via Mesmerism. This psycho-spiritual approach to heightened transpersonal awareness was largely discarded by the Western healing tradition until very recently. This human potential for direct spiritual awareness will be discussed more fully in Chapter 8 on meditation, and Chapters 9-13, on past lives, death, and psychic phenomena.

The somewhat detailed historical survey to be presented here will help lay the conceptual foundation for succeeding chapters, as each therapeutic technique discussed in this book will be shown to impact one layer or dimension in the spectrum of transpersonal experiences. Also, this review will help us to understand the negative bias against hypnosis that permeates American culture. Our children still watch the television cartoon in which Mickey Mouse is hypnotized by the bad guy and forced to do something nefarious to Minnie. The Svengali image created by Hollywood has much to do with hypnosis' low profile among the healing arts. Misunderstanding the difference between Mesmerism and hypnostism, modern clinical science has allowed the taint of Mesmer's flamboyant reputation to be transferred over onto clinical hypnosis, despite the latter being a strictly verbal transaction lacking all of the overt sexualized manipulation that characterized Mesmer's grandiose performances.

Suffice it to say that a revised version of animal magnetism may provide a bridge to understand not only such standard mind/body topics as hypnosis or the relaxation response, but also such controversial and unexplained processes as acupuncture, homeopathy, laying on of hands, and even psychic phenomena. As we acknowledge and access the transpersonal dimensions, previously inexplicable phenomena become understandable.

Mesmer's findings

We turn to Europe in the 1700's, the Age of Enlightenment, when the encrusted dogma of the Catholic church's orthodoxy was slowly being supplanted by scientific discoveries about the fundamental laws of physics and chemistry. Franz Anton Mesmer was born in rural Austria in 1734, but not much is known of his early life.[10] After finishing his medical studies with a thesis about the influence of the planets on human diseases, his marriage to a wealthy Viennese widow in 1767 provided him entrée to the aristocracy in the cultural capital of Europe. He rapidly created a sensation in Vienna with his unorthodox and charismatic treatments of the predominant aristocratic disorders of the day - "les vapeurs" (the vapors) in women, and hypochondriasis in men.

Mesmer used externally applied lodestones (magnets), mysterious hand gestures (the so-called Mesmeric passes) along the length of the patient's body, mirrors, and mechanical equipment to link dozens of patients together for simultaneous treatments. These sessions usually culminated in a healing crisis marked by convulsive laughter, spasmodic jerking of the body (which was embarrassingly sexualized by aristocratic standards), rapid changes in body temperature, fainting spells, and disappearance of symptoms.

Since Mesmer saw himself as part of the European scientific Enlightenment, fighting the dogma and superstition of the Catholic church, he attempted to systematize the working principles of his process by analogy to the physical sciences. He outlined his "27 Principles of Animal Magnetism" (reprinted in Tinterow, see Reference 18), and even patterned his group treatment device, the baquet, after the newly-invented Leyden jar, an electrical capacitor to store electrical charge. He felt that this subtle fluid called animal magnetism interconnected all objects and organisms in the universe, and could be manipulated analogously to the newly discovered force of electricity.

His fame, and his ability to receive generous fees, caused enough concern to the medical establishment that in 1784 a commission of the French Royal Academy under the direction of the American ambassador to France (Benjamin Franklin) investigated Mesmer's work; other leading scientists on the panel included Lavoisier and Guillotine. They concluded, despite having observed only Mesmer's students at work, and never having spoken directly with Mesmer himself, that there was no evidence for the existence of the invisible fluid called animal magnetism, and that any beneficial effects of the treatment (which they did acknowledge to occur) were due solely to suggestion and imagination.[18]

In modern day parlance, we would consider his aristocratic patients to have suffered from functional disorders and conversion symptoms, and so we would not be surprised at their response to nonspecific manipulations of their expectations by a charismatic authority figure. Insightfully, this is what the empirical skeptics of 1784 concluded; they also voiced concern about the potential dangers from the erotic attraction of the magnetized female patient to her male magnetizer. Mesmer was forced to leave Paris, returning to Austria to die without ever having regained his former influence. The taint of charlatanism has stayed with his name, however, despite a repeat French commission in 1831 which vindicated his work.[18]

Interestingly, several of his students continued to practice animal magnetism in France and England, but stripped it of the showmanship and near-hysteria which characterized Mesmer's original work. Of particular note is the work of the British surgeon James Esdaile,[18] who performed major surgery in India in the 1840's using an adaptation of Mesmerism. His technique involved repeated passes of the operator's hands (usually non-Hindi-speaking assistants) along the body of the native Indian patient, often for several hours, without any verbal instruction or cueing, to produce a trance state marked by profound torpor. Several hundred well-documented major surgical procedures were performed (particularly excisions of scrotal hydroceles from endemic parasitic infection), with significantly lower rates of post-surgical complications (infection, hemorrhage and death) than had ever been attained before. His results were in fact superior to the results later obtained under chemical anesthesia (ether and chloroform), but these new chemical techniques rapidly and completely supplanted Mesmerism with their advent in 1845, due to their ease of use and rapid onset of action. Esdaile's well-documented examples of physical healing induced by Mesmeric passes are the precursors of the modern variant of Mesmerism called Therapeutic Touch, to be discussed later.

Mesmer's followers

The French students who followed Mesmer-produced results which are particularly important in understanding the transpersonal states which can be accessed by energy manipulation techniques. Mesmer's disciple Amand-Marie-Jacques de Chastenet, Marquis de Puysegur, was in many ways the opposite to Mesmer. He accepted no fees for his work and he dealt not with the aristocracy but with the peasantry who worked on his familial estate. Several of his cases were written up in some detail and provide a striking contrast with the publicity-conscious frenzy attending Mesmer's soirées. The Marquis de Puysegur initially worked with individual laborers in a calm, low-keyed and respectful manner, and his patients responded without the Mesmeric array of dramatic outbursts. Instead, they entered in a perfect crisis, a state of relaxed attention also called magnetic sleep or artificial somnambulism. The mental lucidity which accompanied this trance allowed for conversations to occur between magnetizer and subject. Strikingly, de Puysegur found that illiterate peasants could make accurate medical diagnoses and prognoses on their own cases. As this practice spread to Germany, it even became common custom to consult so-called somnambulists for health problems and spiritual guidance.[10]

The example of the farmer Victor Race is worth quoting in some detail. Known as the pre-eminent somnambule of his day, he apparently produced medical information far beyond his peasant's ken. Exhibiting what Ellenberger and others described as a dual personality, he was able to make his own medical diagnosis, state the prognosis, and recommend treatments. He even scolded de Puysegur once in a magnetized state, criticizing several recent public demonstrations that brought on a worsening of Race's condition - Mesmerism, he said, was only to be used therapeutically, and not for demonstration or experimentation.

It is interesting that a single technique could produce such widely divergent results, depending on the intent of the therapist and the mindset of the patient. Mesmer's patients were so caught up in their neurotic frivolity that only superficial layers of their psyche were evoked. But it is tempting to conclude that Victor Race and other somnambulists were able to access their higher self or soul through this nondirective technique, perhaps out of transference admiration or imitation of their beloved and exalted patron and magnetizer. It is difficult to ascertain from the historical reports the degree of prompting or unintentional communication between magnetizer and patient, but it seems unlikely that such nonspecific factors could account for such detailed output. Since this type of specialized medical information could certainly not have been learned consciously (or unconsciously) by peasants with no access to higher learning, it seems reasonable to speculate that transpersonal sources of medical information were accessed. Chapter 13, on the process of channelling, will look more closely at this process of accessing information from non-physical sources in the realm of the spirit.

These results also presage and parallel the story of Edgar Cayce, Kentucky's famous Sleeping Prophet of the late 1800's. Cayce was a poorly educated photographer who discovered by accident his ability to enter into a sleep-like trance from which he could give highly detailed medical reports about his own condition. As he came to wider attention, he began to comment on patients whom he had never met before, prescribing a highly complex but consistent series of poultices, herbal remedies, nutritional supplements, and physical and spiritual practices. His vast collection of over 10,000 such readings is now stored at the Edgar Cayce Foundation at the Association for Research and Enlightenbment in Virginia. Interested readers are referred to the works of Sugrue and Stearns for more information on this fascinating chapter of the transpersonal trance in American medicine.

At any rate, Mesmerism soon became a well-established practice that flourished throughout Europe in the early 1800's despite official disapproval. There was a London Mesmeric Infirmary, and a major journal of Mesmerism, *The Zoist*. This journal was edited by the president of the British Medical Association, who was forced to resign his presidency because of his staunch support of animal magnetism.[13] With the rising interest in chemical anesthesia and in biologic medicine, there soon came a complete rejection of these promising variants of Mesmerism, as the new dogma of scientific materialism or reductionism rose to the forefront. This complete disregard of animal magnetism by Western science lasted nearly 200 years until recent work in the emerging field of biomagnetism started to replicate many of these classic findings.

Another British physician, James Braid,[18] completed the transition from Mesmerism to modern clinical hypnosis by stripping away all reference to the alleged magnetic fluidium. In his studies of the fixed attentional focus which characterized the trance state, Braid formulated a neurological theory of trance in 1843, in an essay called "The Physiology of Fascination." He also coined the term "neuro-hypnology," or nervous sleep (hence our modern term hypnosis) to denote the state of receptivity to suggestion which developed when a patient's attention could be fixed and finely focused.

By emphasizing the innate skills of the patient, seeking a neurologic mechanism, rejecting the notion of animal magnetism, and emphasizing the verbal transactions between doctor and patient, Braid laid the foundation for Charcot, Janet, Freud, and modern clinical hypnosis. At the same time, he closed the door of Western medicine on Mesmerism and magnetism. Today, verbal therapies using imagery and suggestion are testimony to the increasing acceptance of the "de-magnetized" version of hypnosis that is pre-eminent today. The popular press today continues to confuse Mesmerism and hypnosis by using the terms synonymously and even in the clinical literature the terms are often not carefully differentiated.

Ironically, then, the Mesmeric brach of clinical hypnosis's family tree is finally coming to fruition now, with modern energy-based treatment like Therapeutic Touch and energy healing (also called the laying on of hands). The latter will be discussed in more detail in Chapter 3, while the former has become so much a part of the curriculum in most American nursing schools over the last twenty years that it is practiced in most hospitals in America today. Developed in the early 1970's by a nurse collaborating with a clairvoyant, this simple treatment is readily learned in a weekend work-shop, and involves developing sensitivity to the fluctuations in a patient's magnetic fluidium, or energy field. It has been perhaps the best researched of the energy therapies, and so provides the link between classic Mesmerism and modern science.

Biomagnetism

The science of biomagnetism today has the high tech ability to investigate electromagnetic phenomena with a precision impossible in past generations. Devices range from simple surface electrode recordings of skin resistance to the sophisticated SQUID (superconducting quantum interference device) measurement of minute fluctuations of the magnetic field. All these devices stem from the commonplace notion that biological activity is fundamentally electrical in nature (i.e., nerve conduction action potentials, muscle contrac-tion, EEG, EKG, etc.), and that moving electrical currents induce a corre-sponding magnetic field that extends out into the surrounding space. So by virtue of our electrically coordinated nervous system symphony, we also generate a pulsating magnetic field surrounding us.

The many exciting discoveries in biomagnetism sound like science fiction. For example, human beings are now known to share with homing pigeons the abilitiy to orient directionally to the earth's magnetic field. We also have a magnetic sensory modality, apparently mediated by a nerve plexus near the ethmoid sinus in the skull that contains magnetite crystals and is disrupt-able by placing a magnet over one's forehead.[1] Highly structured direct cur-rent (DC) electrical field cradients, with their corresponding magnetic fields, have been found to surround and interpenetrate the bodies of all living organisms.[7] These fields appear to correlate with the popularized concepts of personal space and interpersonal distance, and also with the mystical concept of the aura. Similarly, it may be that psychotherapeutic work on boundary issues is not just metaphorical, but may also have an electromagnetic basis that could potentially be measured directly in clinical research.

A brief experiential exercise can help the reader become familiar with the somewhat unusual notion of an energy field surrounding the body.

> Instructions: Begin by rubbing your two hands briskly together for 5 or 10 seconds, and then bring them about two feet apart with the palms facing each other. Begin to move the hands towards each other with a slow, bounding, back and forth movement until they are only an inch apart. Pay attention to the different sensations you notice. Be sure to note the sensation of temperature or warmth transmitted from hand to hand, and distinguish this from the sensation of tingly pressure that becomes evident when the hands are 6 to 12 inches apart.

This last sensation occurs when the edge of the energy field of one hand comes in contact with the outer edge of the field of the other hands. Practice will help you to differentiate this sensation more clearly from the other physical sensations happening at the same time. The size of the gap between the two hands at the moment when the field's edges touch is a measure of the size of your auric field. It widens after exercising, meditating, or simply imagining a flow of energy coursing out of the hands; in context, this gap shrinks when you're tired or sick. Gradation and fluctuation of this magnetic feeling are at the heart of the treatment technique called theapeutic touch.

These magnetic fields also seem to actively direct the processes of cell growth and differentiation, and are not simply indirect side effects of biologic processes. Altering these fields can induce rudimentary limb regeneration in organisms which typically lack this ability.[2] Discrete areas of increased electrical conductivity on the skin have recently been found which exactly match the location of classic Chinese acupuncture points,[2] suggesting that the Chinese model of acupuncture with its points and meridians is not simply a cultural superstition, but is rather the outcome of centuries of careful introspection and clinical experience. Even the placement by today's pain specialists of transcutaneous electrical nerve stimulator (TENS) electrodes on acupuncture points is at least a grudging acknowledgement by Western medicine that something important is going on here.

Sleep, and anesthesia, can be rapidly induced in salamanders by applying external magnets;[2] reversing the polarity of the magnet reverses the physical effect. This suggests that changes in consciousness are not chemically mediated, as it is in surgical anesthesia via inhaled anesthetics or in medication treatment of insomnia. Perhaps there is also an unexplored biomagnetic mechanism linking mind to magnetic field. Perhaps magnetic anesthesia for surgery may return (Mesmerists in the operating room), as might the use of external electrical currents to facilitate healing (now used by orthopedists to heal pathologic bone fractures).

During altered states of consciousness such as meditation or healing, the external magnetic field of a subject changes. Preliminary studies with SQUID[16] have begun, but funding difficulties have prevented further research with SQUID. Some studies suggest that hypnotic suggestion may also work by a biomagnetic process, wherein regional changes in electromagnetic potential can be induced by suggestion. For example, a hypnotically anesthetized limb is accompanied by measurable changes in the DC current in the brain of the subject.[12]

This electromagnetic mechanism may explain how certain psychiatric conversion disorders (marked by the development of pseudo-neurologic symptoms like blindness or deafness, without any nerve damage) don't follow standard anatomic patterns, leading to numb hands or pain in the feet, even though human nerve pathways don't follow this pathway by ending at the wrist or ankle. Rather, there may be a form of self-hypnosis at work in generating these functional conversion symptoms. Perhaps hypnotic suggestions can alter specific regions of the body's electromagnetic field according to the particular imagery held in the patient's mind; the neurologic pathways can be bypassed by these electromagnetic fluxes. As the mystics said, energy follows thought, and physiology follows energy; perhaps electromagnetic fields are the mediators of these puzzling forms of energy transformation.

A modern variant of Mesmerism called Therapeutic Touch is being taught as part of the standard nursing school curriculum to thousands of RN's in America today. This technique also involves noncontact passes of the hands along the length of the patient's body and has been demonstrated to speed up the process of wound healing (see Reference 19, an extremely well-controlled scientific experiment) and to enhance the growth of premature infants in a neonatal intensive care unit.[14] In both studies, nonspecific expectancy effects were controlled for, eliminating placebo and hypno-suggestive factors. Therapeutic Touch has had to endure its own Royal Commission, with the recent notorious attempt to discount and debunk it in the *Journal of the American Medical Association.* for a critique of the article, see Reference 15b. Much has been written about direct hands-on approach to healing,[5,6] and these phenomena also seem to be electromagnetically mediated. Chapter 3 will deal with the transpersonal trance aspects of hands on healing in greater detail. Clearly, further measurement of the DC fields and SQUID events accompanying these hypno-therapeutic processes will be crucial to validate this energy field model.

Another intriguing aspect of electromagnetic fields is that they can interact with one another by a process of resonance, much like tuning forks which vibrate in tandem. This process could explain how high-voltage transmission lines might induce human disease, by an entrainment process called biomagnetic resonance[2] that is mediated by electromagnetic fields rather than by direct radiation. Of interest to psychiatrists is a 30-year-old report which correlates psychiatric hospitalization rates with fluctuations in the earth's magnetic field.[12] The phase of the moon has been disproved as the signal generator (despite popular notions about "lunatics"), suggesting a process of magneto-behavioral resonance rather than one of direct astrological influence (or maybe astrology is mediated by differing magnetic fields set up by the planets).

Finally, it has been speculated that clinical intuitions and hunches are a resonance phenomenon between the tuning forks of the therapist's and the patient's interacting electromagnetic fields. Particularly empathic therapists may simply have learned how to allow their emotional tuning forks to resonate in an unrestricted manner, while cold or distant clinicians may have clamped down their oscillation to the point where no interaction is percieved. Chapter 4 by John Tatum will explore this possibility in further detail.

The notion of "life energy" which pervades all non-Western healing traditions[15] may have its roots in subtle bioelectric phenomena of the sorts outlined above. This field metaphor is quite fascinating and intuitively seductive, so hopefully more research will emerge to ascertain the validity of these images. The tests need be no more complex than to measure the strength and extent of these fields in radiantly healthy people (notice how our common figures of speech reflect this model), and compare them with the fields of severely ill people.

Case study

A clinical vignette can illustrate the power of the energy field metaphor: Anthony was a 26 year-old man who worked as a stock boy on the night shift at a local warehouse because his schizotypal personality style prevented him from flourishing in any setting that required frequent contact with other people. He described his constant sense of carrying his father's strict criticisms in his own mind, as though they were actual objects inside his head. He also was extremely sensitive to his father's physical presence and felt frightened and guilt-ridden simply when in his vicinity. Anthony was maintained on low doses of antipsychotic medicines because he often found it difficult to disengage from these troublesome thoughts and was often unable to distinguish whether they were internal or external.

He was taught an imagery process that allowed him to create a zone of light and clarity and safety around him, surrounded by a semipermeable protective membrane that would only let in influences which he decided were useful to him. He was encouraged to practice this visualization in each of his main life settings, to develop the sense that he was concretely in control of his own emotional boundaries. He reported becoming less sensitive to these previously upsetting external influences. Although he did not significantly increase his ability to socialize, he was less troubled by his father's introjected thoughts and feeling, and he began to feel more in control of his own inner experiences and less vulnerable to the impact of other people.

In other words, Anthony was able to use the metaphor of the human energy aura in a way that was protective and empowering for him. He was able to sharpen his psychotically permeable boundaries, and to place outside of his field certain intrusive and critical ideas.

So clinically, anecdotally and experientially, the field metaphor seems useful. However, the validity of the research data to back up these claims may be questioned. Close inspection of the accompanying bibliography will show that the key studies which have been completed to date on energy medicine have generally not been published in preeminent medical journals. However, this may be as much a political issue as a question of methodological rigor and scientific validity. Organized science appears to resist paradigm-threatening data as forcefully today as it did in Mesmer's era. Certain exceptions[8,17] prove the rule.

The publication of each of these two articles became a "cause celèbre" for the journal, involving (expecially in the former case) the adoption of far more stringent review criteria than was normally used for non-controversial reports. They also allowed a skeptical and hostile witness to observe the replication of the original study. For a description of the difficulties in obtaining institutional support and government funding for work in these controversial areas, the postscript of Robert Becker's book *Cross Currents* is illuminating. Perhaps the recent formation by the NIH of an Office of Alternative Medicine, and the launching of such new medical journals as the *Journal of Alternative Therapies*, will reverse this tendency. Of necessity I've cited some fairly obscure journals, but I've also included details of how to obtain reprints, so readers can judge for themselves the quality of the work referenced here.

Conclusion

In summary, it seems quite possible that mind and body may interact through the mediation of electromagnetic fields. Today's clinical hypnosis may involve verbally induced shifts in the energy field, while Mesmeric variants may involve shifts directed specifically at the energy field itself, without verbal mediation. And when the energy field shifts, the body follows suit. Thus, we must be careful not to repeat the mistake of the Franklin Commission in 1784 that created a political climate hostile to any further scientific study of animal magnetism. There appears to be enough wheat of solid experimental and clinical data among the chaff of wild unproven claims to justify an unbiased exploration of the scientific underpinnings of these unusual phenomena. This continued scientific exploration of previously ignored territory may soon radically expand our understanding of human consciousness and its relation to health and disease, and thus bring about a crucial paradigm shift. And hypnosis will prove to be a key tool for accessing these transpersonal domains.

References:

1. Baker, R.R., Human Magnetoreception for Navigation, in *Electromagnetic Fields and Neurobehavioral Function*, O'Connor and Lovely, Eds., Alan Liss, New York, 1988.
2. Becker, R. et al., Clinical experiences with low intensity direct current stimulation of bone growth, in *Clinical Orthopedics and Related Research*, 124:75, 1977.
3. Becker, Robert, *Cross Currents: the perils of electropollution and the promise of electromedicine*, J. Tarcher, Los Angeles, 1988.
4a. Braid, James, The physiology of fascination, in *Foundation of Hypnosis*, M. Tinterow, Ed., Charles Thomas, Springfield, IL, 1970.
4b. Braid, James, Neurypnology, in *Foundation of Hypnosis*, M. Tinterow, Ed., Charles Thomas, Inc., 1970.
5. Bruyere, Rosalyn, *Wheels of Light*, Simon & Schuster, New York, 1989.
6. Brennan, Barbara, *Hands of Light*, Bantam, New York, 1991.
7. Burr, Harold Saxton, *Blueprint for immortality: the electric patterns of life*, Neville Spearman Ltd., London, 1972.
8. Davenas, E., et al., Human basophil degranulation triggered by ver dilute antiserum against IgAE, *Nature*, 333:816–818, 1988.
9. Eisenberg, D., et al., Unconventional Medicine in the United States: prevalence, cost, patterns of use, *New England J. Med.*, 328, 4, 246–252, 1993.
10. Ellenberger, Henri, *The Discovery of the Unconscious*, Basic Books, New York, 1970.
11. Friedman, H., et al., Direct current potential in hypnoanalgesia, *Arch. Gen. Psychiatry*, 7:193, 1962.
12. Friedman, H. et al., Geomagnetic Parameters and Psychiatric Hospital Admissions, *Nature*, 200:4907, 626–628, Nov. 16, 1963.
13. Gauld, A., Reflections of Mesmeric analgesia, *Br. J. Experimental and Clin. Hypnosis*, 5:1, 17–24, 1988.
14. Krieger, D., Therapeutic Touch: the imprimatur of nursing, *Amer. J. Nursing*, 75:784–787, 1975.
15. Leskowitz, E., Life energy and western medicine: a reappraisal, *Advances*, 8:1, 63–67, 1992.
15b. Leskowitz, E., Un-debunking my Therapeutic Touch, *Alternative Therapies*, www.alternative-therapies.com.
16. New Technologies Detect Effects of Healing Hands, *Brain/Mind Bulletin*, 7:3, Sept. 30, 1985, PO Box 42211, Los Angeles.
17. Rosa, A closer look a Therapeutic Touch, JAMA.
18. Tart, Charles et al., Information Transmission in Remote Viewing Experiments, *Nature*, 284(5752):1911, 13 March 1980.
19. Tinterow, M., Ed., *Foundations of Hypnosis*, Charles Thomas Inc., Springfield, IL, 1970.
20. Wirth, Daniel, The Effect of Noncontact Therapeutic Touch on the Healing Rate of Full Thickness Dermal Wounds, *Subtle Energy*, 1:1, 1–20, 1990.
21. Zimmerman, John, Laying-On of Hands Healing and Therapeutic Touch: A Testable Theory, in *The Newsletter of the Bio-Electro-Magnetics Institute*, 2:1, 1990.

For further study:

Therapeutic Touch training
Pumpkin Hollow Farm
Rt. 11
Craryville, NY 12521
(518) 325-3583
email: Pumpkin@taconic.net

Nurse Healer's Association
P.O.Box 444
Allison Park, PA 15101-0444
(414) 355-8476

chapter three

Energy healing and hypnosis

Eric D. Leskowitz

Introduction

The laying on of hands is probably the oldest method of relieving suffering and healing illnesses devised by man, yet it is also one of the least understood. With roots going back to Biblical times in our Western tradition, and even further back in some Eastern cultures, it is obvious that humanity has long been interested in the power of human touch.[1] Today, with a growing interest in alternative or holistic approaches to health care, there is also an increase in the number of practitioners who claim to be able to heal by touch. Thus, it is important to understand this practice. Does it simply involve religious superstition and placebo factors? Is it a hypnosuggestive trance state? Can it be justifiably integrated into modern Western medicine? As an American trained physician who practices the laying on of hands (in the non-sectarian form known as energy healing), I offer my perspective on this important topic.

In this chapter, I'll expand on the model of the human energy field introduced in Chapter 2, and show how the unique conjoint trance of energy healing allows transpersonal dimensions of consciousness to be directly accessed and experienced by both the patient and the healer. This healing technique is not simply a matter of mechanically manipulating biomagnetic life energy (as in acupuncture, for example), because it also involves a particular state of focused attention by both subject and healer that is in effect a mutual hypnotic trance. Because aspects of Self from the spiritual realms are invoked and accessed, energy healing should rightly be categorized as a transpersonal trance state, rather than as a simple energy manipulation technique.

The term *to heal* deserves special consideration at the outset, especially as it will be used in contrast to the more limited medical term *to cure*, which means to make physical symptoms go away without regard for underlying causes. Healing originates from the Old English word *haelen* meaning *to heal*; it is also related with the words *health* and *holy* and *whole*. So wholeness, health, and holiness are linked in our linguistic unconscious, as these etymologies presage our supposedly modern discussions about spirituality and health, and the multidimensional nature of man. As I'll discuss below, medical curing is only one dimensional, but man can only become whole when his physical, emotional, cognitive, and spiritual dimensions are all included and embraced.

In this chapter, I'll begin by reviewing the history of energy healing (those aspects not already discussed in the chapter on animal magnetism), and then I'll review evidence which helps us to reconceptualize many unusual psychospiritual events as the result of changes in the human energy field. Several case vignettes will be presented, and then some speculation and suggestions for future research will all be outlined in a manner which synthesizes the apparently unrelated phenomena of hypnotic trance and energy healing. This discussion will include more metaphor and analogy than hard fact, but it will present some exciting images for the reader to consider in assessing his or her own energetic experiences in everyday life.

The history of energy healing

For many people looking at the topic of energy healing and the laying on of hands, its strong religious connotation is discouraging. This ambivalence arises in two ways. First, people may respond to the stories of Biblical healing at the hands of such masters as Jesus or St. Paul and say, "Well, those are such highly evolved beings that I cannot possibly hope to experience something like that myself." Alternatively, people of a more skeptical (scientific), agnostic or atheistic bent may feel that these Biblical reports are simply inaccurate legends, embellished by 2000 years of uncritical repetition; any modern derivatives of this practice must therefore be built on a foundation of sand. Because these two thought patterns are so prevalent in America today, many contemporary Americans are ready to dismiss energy healing outright, without consideration of the available scientific and historical evidence.

Actually, in the European tradition, there have been many non-Biblical and even non-religious practitioners of this art. The British monarchs were traditionally believed to have the healing touch, as an offshoot of their divine rights, and commoners were often allowed to experience the royal touch as a medical treatment in and of itself.

Commoners too had this ability: consider, for example, John Greatrakes, the well-known country healer of Shakespeare's era.[2] But after the fall of Mesmerism and animal magnetism almost 200 years ago, the Western tradition of energy healing went into hibernation. Mesmerism evolved into the "de-magnetized" technique of clinical hypnosis, which used focused attention and verbal suggestions to bring about psychological and physiological changes without any manipulation by touch of the alleged "magnetic fluidium."

Luckily, the Eastern life energy techniques have continued to be actively practiced for millennia, in China as external Qi Gong and in India as Prana Massage. The Western renaissance of energy healing over the past 30 years draws from these cross-cultural roots, as evoked by such current treatment names as: Reiki, Shiatsu, Pranic Healing, Therapeutic Touch, Kahuna Healing, Bioplasm Therapy, etc. The heuristic model which many contemporary energy healers use to explain their work incorporates elements from both the Indian and Chinese schools, and so it is worth detouring for a moment into the finer points of the Eastern energy model to understand exactly how human energetics is involved in both energy healing and the trance state. This will help us to understand how hypnotic trances work , and how they may so readily access transpersonal realms of experience.

Human subtle anatomy

The basic notion here is that human beings are multidimensional organisms, not simply pieces of physical machinery. We possess a gross physical anatomy, as well as a subtle energetic anatomy. The former is dissected in the pathology lab, the latter in the meditation retreat. In the yogic version of this concept, these levels of vibrational structure are called koshas, *sheaths*.[3] The physical body is called the food sheath, because it is composed of rearranged food components. This name is in itself a quite powerful reframing of our beliefs about who we really are. You'e *not* what you eat. Your physical body is what you eat, but you are more than just a physical body. The next most subtle layer is called the energy or breath sheath (pranamaya kosha) because it is composed of an organized network of prana energy derived from our breath. Though most ordinary people are not able to directly perceive this sheath, it is considered in Yoga to be nearly as dense as the physical body itself. Then there is the layer of emotions (known in the West as the astral body), and then a layer of thoughts (the mental body), and finally the highest frequency layer of spiritual essence (the causal body, or soul).

Chinese medicine tends to focus primarily on the pranic sheath, the densest of these subtle layers. It manipulates the prana or qi (also spelled chi) via acupuncture needles to help this energy flow freely through the body's distribution network that we know as the acupuncture meridians. Tai chi (movement) and qi gong (imagery) are other major methods of enhancing this energy flow. Both are clearly trance-like in nature, as practitioners become absorbed in a state of complete internal focus. Yoga philosophy also recognizes these same meridians (calling them *nadis*), and cleanses them through specialized breathing techniques and imagery meditations which focus and direct the flow of energy to desired regions of the body. This breath technology will be discussed further in Chapter 6; it can directly alter hemispheric activation patterns and induce trance phenomena nonverbally simply by regulating the flow of prana.

By analogy, we could use the language of physics to say that human beings are composed of several layers of varying density. Just as H_2O can exist as a solid (ice), a liquid (water), or a gas (steam), depending on the rate of thermal vibration of its H_2O molecules, so our physical bodies are condensed and solid in nature, while our emotional and mental bodies are more liquefied, and our purest spiritual awareness is vapor-like and insubstantial. But all three dimensions are still different forms of the same underlying element: pure consciousness.

In India more than China, great importance was also placed on the major distribution centers within this network of nested energy bodies. These energy centers were called *chakras*, or wheels, and are involved with the absorption, transformation, and distribution of this universal pranic energy. Their locations have been systematized over the centuries only on the basis of meditative experiences and introspection, since no gross anatomical dissection was allowed in the Hindu tradition. Western physicians have only recently discovered a series of striking correspondences between the location of these subjective energy centers and the anatomic structures known as endocrine glands.[4]

The small ductless endocrine glands, seem to be exact parallels in structure and function to the chakras, and may serve as the transducers which take life energy of varying frequencies and convert it into biochemical signals of the appropriate order (i.e., the hormone products that are made by each endocrine gland). The accompanying chart (Figure 3.1) shows some of the correspondences between endocrine gland, hormone product, energy center, and dominant emotional frequency. Again, the multidimensional nature of this spectrum is key.

Chakra	#	Gland	Color	Emotion	Sensation	Drug
Crown	7	Pineal	Violet	Bliss	tingling scalp	psychedelics
Brow	6	Pituitary	Indigo	Insight	"light bulb"	psychedelics, THC
Throat	5	Thyroid	Blue	Truth	choked-up	alcohol
Heart	4	Thymus	Green	Love	warm-hearted	MDMA
Solar Plexus	3	Pancreas	Yellow	Power	"butterflies"	alcohol, THC
Genital	2	Gonads	Orange	Sexuality	arousal	alcohol, THC
Root	1	Adrenals	Red	Survival	"adrenaline rush"	cocaine

Figure 3.1 Energy center correspondences.

It is amazing that introspection was accurate enough to assign these seven centers to the same bodily locations that medieval anatomists discovered centuries later. Even the location of several endocrine glands whose functions were considered mysterious if not vestigial until recently (the pineal gland and the thymus) fits in cleanly with the chakra model. But even more intriguing is the notion that a psychospiritual function is associated with each center, in a hierarchy from the lower centers (which deal with physical survival) to the higher centers (which modulate refined emotions like love and bliss). Again, there is the sense that each major emotion has an energetic frequency: the lower or coarser emotions of selfishness have a lower vibration than the selfless ones of truth and love. That is why colors have also been assigned to each center in Figure 3.1, as another way of reinforcing the spectrum or continuum view of consciousness: a range of vibrational frequencies running from pure unitary consciousness to dense physical matter. Einstein's $e = mc^2$ becomes the mathematical restatement of this interconvertibility of spiritual energy and matter.

Some of the recently discovered biochemical functions of the endocrine glands are eerily reminiscent of the ancient mystical functions ascribed to the chakras. These functional correspondences actually help to validate the chakra model by being so statistically unlikely. For example, it is not difficult to ascribe sexual feelings to the genital areas, as even the most non-introspective person has felt the rush of erotic life energy to this area during times of arousal. Why, though, is it so common to describe the sensation of sudden insight as a light bulb going off inside one's head; why is an upsurge of love felt behind the sternum; why is fear felt as butterflies in the stomach? The heart beats faster in fear, therefore a simple somatic referent would locate fear to the heart, too.

I believe that these linguistic idioms contain a deep proprioceptive wisdom because they capture subtle but commonplace energetic experiences that corroborate the chakra map. The image of a light bulb of intuition is the modern description of the opening of the mystic third eye; heartwarming love is the 4th chakra opening; butterflies in the stomach area is a sudden rush of 3rd chakra energy for personal power.

And consider the biologic functions of each center. Personal power is collected in the gut (the hara, in martial arts), just as pancreatic insulin from this same solar plexus area helps us to collect the glucose that biochemically fuels all our physical actions. Adrenaline's fight or flight survival reaction is triggered by activation of a root chakra that generates energy for physical survival. The mystic enlightenment that comes with an open crown chakra parallels recent work on circadian rhythms: the pineal gland is now known to translate day/night sunlight rhythms into hormone fluctuations, and therefore links each individual to the rhythms of the solar system, just as the ancients took enlightenment to be a merger of the individual with the universe.

This detailed outline of subtle anatomy has not been a detour from our original topic since it underlies both energy healing and hypnosis by explaining their mechanism of action. But in order to connect these two therapies by an energy-based mechanism, we need to propose a method of energy transfer. For that, we turn to the coupled oscillation of two vibrating objects: resonance. A familiar example is how one tuning fork will vibrate in sympathy with another struck fork; an open guitar string vibrates in response to a sung musical note of the same pitch or frequency. Our language even has many idiomatic expressions for a similar kind of resonance between feelings or thoughts: an idea rings a bell, a person has a nice vibe, two people are on the same wavelength, a stranger's entreaty can strike a sympathetic chord. We all know the resonance process by which emotions are spread: a conference room can be contaminated by the anger of one forceful member, laughter is contagious, and a group can rise to the heights of an inspirational leader. These images all "ring true" because they reflect our unconscious understanding that awareness is a field of resonant energy.

Significantly, vibratory frequencies can also be carried by physical structures in the body. Some cellular components (i.e., intracellular microtubules) actually look like tiny resonant tuning forks, while some tissue structures (i.e., the bone matrix and the collagen in connective fascia) have an electrical and crystalline nature that can transmit resonant frequencies. Researchers have even postulated that bones function via piezo-electricity,[5] much like a crystal radio set that converts the physical micromovements of sound waves into electromagnetic waves by its piezo-electric crystals. Similarly, when a person walks, the mechanical strain on the bones causes the hydroxy-apatite biocrystals in the bony matrix to transmit tiny electrical currents. These microcurrents then function as informational signals that regulate the bone's growth and structural formation. In a similar way, each region of the body will electromagnetically resonate at the frequency of its nearest chakra, the overall keynote for each bodily region.

A diseased organ may become uncoupled from its healthy natural maintenance frequency in many ways: by exposure to toxins, stress (for example, the low frequency vibration of constant fear), poor nutrition, etc. But an organ can become healthy again if it is exposed to the matrix energy of a healthy organ. This does not mean that an ailing stomach can be healed by placing it near a healthy one. Rather, if the stomach's energy blueprint can be re-primed to vibrate at the proper energetic frequency, then the physical outgrowth or manifestation of this subtle energy field will be a newly healthy organ. Remember that the physical structures of the body are believed to be the solid precipitation of matter in alignment with the subtle organizing electromagnetic fields,[6] just as the iron filings aligned with the bar magnet's lines of force in a school science lab. Rupert Sheldrake's abstract notion of preformative morphogenetic fields may have their physical foundation in this type of biomagnetism.[7]

Thus, if the body's electromagnetic energy field becomes disordered, the correlated organ will soon follow suit and manifest a physical disease. This might explain the claim that the onset of physical illness can be predicted by antecedent change in the energy aura, detected by Kirlian photography or clairvoyant perception. If energy really does follow thought, as the mystics say, then no one will be surprised to learn that most diseases can have emotional roots, since negative emotions block the full force of broad spectrum life energy. Energy healing can be seen as a process in which the healer brings about sympathetic resonance between his own finely tuned body/mind energetic system and that of the patient. The healer himself becomes the instrument of healing. And one of the most important steps that can enhance this resonant energy exchange between two people is the state of focused attentiveness we call hypnosis.

Energetic aspects of hypnosis

Hypnotherapy at its most profound is an interaction between two people who have each entered a state of deep absorption. A therapist who simply recites a rote hypnotic induction script does not create the deep healing states that occur when the hypnotherapist also allows himself to become entranced in the process. Then, a therapist can become receptive to exquisitely subtle feedback from the patient, not simply the depth of respiration or level of muscle tension that are hallmarks of light trance in traditional hypnosis, but also unconscious, even psychic, cues of thought, feeling, and intention. Let us now consider several types of energy field interaction that may underlie these unusual hypnotic phenomena.

· Startling intuitive insights involving specific information not transmitted by the five physical senses are often experienced by hypnotherapists, and have been described by authors from Jung[8] to Tart.[9] When a therapist becomes aware of his own internal subtle energetic processes, he is able to resonantly detect changes occuring in his patient's energy field, especially when empathy is complete, and there is a merger of the two fields. An example of such a psychic or transpersonal insight occured in my office practice recently.

I was preparing myself for my next patient's appointment by consciously making myself receptive to any intuitive information that might be availabe about him, and I mentally reviewed our recent work together. Nothing specific came to me during this light daydream, but as I heard his car pull into the parking lot outside my office window, I had a sudden vivid image of an oak tree just before I returned to normal waking consciousness. I initially dismissed this picture as random or irrelevant mental garbage, until my patient sat down and began to talk. His very first words described his recent decision to move back to his native land of Israel, because he felt his roots were there, he was close to the land there, and he felt unconnected to the earth in America. He had spontaneously compared himself to a tree, before I'd had a chance to say anything at all.

Perhaps my empathic connection to him had allowed me to resonantly pick up on his current emotionally (and therefore energetically) charged preoccupation. Recent experimental work documents specific brainwave correlations that occur when two people experience this subjective state of merger.[10] This receptive aspect of the therapist's trance, discussed further in Chapter 4 on empathy, represents only one use of the entranced therapist's heightened energy awareness.

A pro-active alteration of therapist energy states is possible, and affects the patient's trance process even more directly than this responsive empathy. Remember that the therapist in trance can also actively manipulate his own energy field state (via imagery or intention), to bring about a desired resonance effect on the patient's energy field, and thereby on his trance experience. The therapist can choose to engender a helpful new frequency by setting a new emotional tone within himself, and allowing resonant induction to bring this experience to the patient nonverbally.

So the energy field view of trance phenomena holds that the therapist establishes a dominant emotional frequency via his own personal state of being, as modified by the power dynamics of the treatment relationship. This process occurs in all relationships, to be sure, but in therapy it is consciously manipulated for the patient's benefit. And larger group fields correspondingly establish more powerful group trances, whether it's the coherent field of a finely tuned organization (a choir, a corporation, or a baseball team), or the shared fervor of sports fans. This revealing word, *fan*, is short for fanatic, from the Latin *fanum*, meaning temple, and *fanaticus*, god-inspired; it is also cognate with *profane*. Another method of helping a patient learn about a new frequency or feeling-state is by allowing it to emerge spontaneously from within the unconscious or higher self of the patient, as demonstrated in Chapter 7 by the Personal Totem Pole imagery process.

In order to explain the efficacy of hypnotic suggestions, we turn to another metaphor, the mind as a radio. Different states of awareness (alertness, daydreaming, deep sleep, etc.) are seen as different stations on the radio band, which allow you to access different types of information. Hypnosis is allowing someone else to have temporary control over your tuning dial, and therapeutic suggestion is the process by which someone else sets the tuning dial of your awareness at a new frequency. These suggestions may be benign, as when the vibe of optimism or self-confidence is substituted for self-criticism or depression. But new frequencies can also be hypnotically implanted in unconscious and manipulative ways as in television advertising.

When a television viewer becomes hypnotically transfixed in front of the set, the advertisements create dissatisfaction and implant suggestions to buy new products to attain happiness. Similarly, the mass media's preoccupation with tragedy and violence induces a "victim" trance of fear and helplessness in its viewers. This mindset can be paralyzing, and can engender the same sort of learned helplessness seen in post-traumatic stress disorder (PTSD). The energy healer Rosalyn Bruyere uses the evocative phrase "trauma trance" to describe the mechanism that underlies this process of induced victimization.

In effect, the energy field of the therapist *is* the trance induction, and the words are secondary. Whoever has the biggest aura wins. The therapist's words affect the digitally oriented left cerebral hemisphere, while his energy field affects the analog, DC current-responsive right hemisphere (see Becker's model of the dual nervous system[11]). Each human being can potentially resonate to any frequency if their chakras are suitably unblocked. An inspiring therapist can bring in experiences from the higher domains, and thereby introduce the patient to new frequencies of experience.

Charisma takes on a new meaning when viewed through the lens of energy field manipulation. It becomes easier to understand how one speaker can pull a crowd in his direction when we realize that personal magnetism is not simply a figure of speech but a literal reality. Masters of crowd manipulation like Hitler not only chose the most potent imagery and language in their speeches, but they also knew (consciously or unconsciously) how to work with energy fields by harmonizing and integrating the diverse individual fields into one coherent group field which could actually take on a life of its own.[12] Whether used benevolently, as in a passionate religious sermon, or for evil intent via political manipulation, the underlying process is the same. According to the classic definition of magic as the use of ritual and ceremony to harness energy, white magic uses this energy for good and black magic for evil. Notice also the role of music in both cases, to set the tone with pounding martial beat, or with stirring gospel melodies. Another vibration at work.

Meditation can be reexamined in this light, as a technique which allows one to disengage from dominant frequencies (i.e., internal dialog, bodily preoccupations, and limiting cultural beliefs) and to thereby be opened to higher non-egoic frequency selection. As Wolinsky states in Chapter 8, meditation allows us to 'de-hypnotize' ourselves from the trances we live, rising naturally to the highest altitude/frequency domain. In the form of meditation known as Shabd Yoga, the mantra is actually seen as an internal sound focus chosen to register at a certain vibrational harmonic that is most beneficial for the student.

Energy healing as a trance state

We have so far considered the non-specific effect that one person's overall field has on another, or what has been called the radiatory type of energy healing by presence.[13] Another more specific and focused use of the human energy field occurs in the various hands-on healing approaches like laying on of hands, Reiki and external Qi Gong. I will now discuss a healing approach that uses the specific biomagnetic qualities of the healer to alter the patient's bodily processes. This energy healing builds on the foundation of the healers radiatory healing presence, and then allows for additional specific magnetic manipulations of chosen aspects of the energy field. The shared transpersonal trance of the merged energy fields then enables information to be accessed from physical, emotional, mental, and spiritual levels.

In this approach, as taught by Barbara Brennan,[14] Rosalyn Bruyere[15] and others, the healer engages in an active imagery process as part of his own inner trance work. In its most generalized form, the healer cultivates an image of sunlight coming into his body from a universal source, and shining out from the palms of both hands, which are then placed on the affected body parts of the patient.

Interestingly, in numerous workshop experiences, I've noticed that the volunteer patient can generally perceive a change in sensation when the healer begins to imagine the flow of energy moving through his hands into the patient. This accords with research findings that patients can subjectively differentiate between sham and real therapeutic touch in a controlled research setting.[16] Further proof that this is not simply an exercise in suggestion comes from work with energy healing for plants and animals, exhaustively documented by Benor.[17]

The color or frequency of this light energy is adjusted with imagery to match the physiologic needs of the patient, in accordance with a model that is partly empiric and partly intuitive. For example, in the treatment of acute pain, a cool blue color is typically felt by patients to be most soothing; this makes sense intuitively (blue = water = cool = numb). For reasons that are not obvious, neurologic injuries seem to respond best to gold frequencies. Each healer has a unique way of perceiving and interpreting the energetic input from patients, some perceive in the classic clairvoyant visual manner to see colors or structures while other hear different tones or simply "feel" different proprioceptive qualities. Some healers rely totally on intuition to establish a treatment plan, as the session unfolds; others claim to receive information from seemingly external sources regarding the nature of the patients condition, in accord with the channelling phenomenon described further in Chapter 13.

Two vignettes from my clinical practice will illustrate one approach to this process of hypnotically assisted energy healing. I hope the examples will show how energy field manipulations and hypnotic trance processes interdigitate. As backgound, many of my patients have been in extensive rehabilitation for chronic pain problems. They are dealing with the chronic pain, disability, and depression left over from injuries and accidents many years ago. I often start my work with them by doing traditional talk psychotherapy. Since there is always a great emotional cost to loss of the job function and self-esteem, this standard talk therapy can be quite useful.

But then the physical dimension must be linked to these emotional or cognitive issues. For example, many patients have become so absorbed in the sensations coming from the painful part of their body that most of their attention during the day is involved in fighting against these uncomfortable feelings; this leaves them feeling drained of energy. I will invite the patient to explore the feelings more closely, to get to know this so-called inner enemy. Using simple imagery and internal body scanning techniques, it is often possible to bring about major shifts in the pain level, which lead to major improvements in daily functioning. For interested patients, I will next add the dimension of energy healing.

This process usually looks something like a physical therapy session, with the patient lying face up (fully clothed) on a doctor's examining table. I will take a moment to collect my own thoughts and center myself in the intent to be of service to the patient. Then I will place my hands lightly over the major chakras. I leave my hands in each position for a few moments, as I imagine that a stream of light is flowing out of my hands into the patient's body. I let the patient feel free to notice any sensations that may arise. Sometimes the process is fairly streamlined, with the patient quiet and reporting nothing more than a feeling of deep ease and comfort. At other times, feelings or memories come into the patient's awareness that are connected in some way to the part of the body that we are focusing on, and it is during the ensuing dialog that things get interesting. Let me give an example.

Case study

Ms. A was a 41-year-old nurse with a three year history of lower back pain that developed gradually because she had been in poor physical condition after a series of flare-ups in her chronic intestinal disease (Crohn's disease); she had also become dependent on pain killing medications. She responded well to an intensive inpatient pain management program, weaning gradually from the narcotic medications, using physical therapy to regain her aerobic fitness, using biofeedback to learn how to control her own unconscious muscle tension, and using group therapy to begin to talk for the first time about the fears and frustrations that went with her chronic medical conditions.

I saw her initially for supportive psychotherapy to help her through this challenging course of treatment. However, she became very involved in learning more about the family origins of her self-defeating attitudes, and we began weekly psychotherapy. Her abdominal condition flared up again during the course of this process, and she asked whether there was some way to focus the deep relaxation skills she'd learned onto her particular problem organ, the intestine. She agreed to try the hands on healing technique, and we were soon able to quiet down acute intestinal attacks through a combination of her own ability to visualize inner healing, and through the regular application of healing energy to the abdomen, which she perceived as a soothing cool blue light that replaced the fiery red pockets of inflammation. She went on to enjoy the longest period of her adult life without relapse of her Crohn's disease.

Also, when she learned to focus her attention without fear on her abdomen during our work, she was able to spontaneously remember a previously forgotten assault that occured when she was 10. This trauma happened a few weeks before the first full-scale flare-up of her intestinal symptoms. The terror and helplessness she felt during the trauma was focused in the same region, the abdomen, where her medical symptoms eventually developed. She was first able to remember the intense butterflies in her stomach, and this feeling served as a bridge to remembering the event itself. The soothing energy feelings helped her both to disengage from this painful memory and to give voice to the stifled emotions of that moment (which she had never told anyone about). Since healing this memory, and the behavior pattern of feeling helpless and victimized that resulted from it, she was able to return to regular work for the first time in four years.

Our sessions usually lasted 45 minutes, about half of the time spent in actual hands on work, and we met almost weekly for over one year to attain this level of emotional and physical healing. In this case, there was a dramatic connection between the woman's emotional state and her physical state, as her body seemed to remember an event which she had consciously forgotten. Even though her bowel disease is thought of by doctors as an organic physical problem, the energy work enabled her to experience this mind/body connection more effectively than simple talk therapy, and I believe that it greatly sped up her overall healing process. She has chosen not to undergo the uncomfortable diagnostic tests which would show whether her intestinal tissue has been restored to normal, and while this information would make for a neater clinical demonstration, I respected her wishes and did not urge her to change her mind.

Another vignette demonstrates how energy awareness can catalyze the psychotherapeutic process, even if no specific physical healing occurs, thus reminding us of the close connection between emotions and energy.

Case study

The patient was a 33-year old construction worker whose leg had been crushed in a work site accident, necessitating an above-the-knee amputation. He developed stump pain and phantom limb pain which prevented him from performing any sort of adapted work. He lost no time in any sort of emotional reaction to the loss, and his high level of motivation convinced his worker's compensation insurance carrier to cover more rehab services than they traditionally did. His metropolitan newspaper wrote a human interest story documenting his frustrations with the medical system.

His pain was unresponsive to the usual array of painkillers and neuro-pathic stabilizing medications, as well as to traditional physical therapy measures. Out of desperation, he agreed to a trial of therapeutic touch. We discovered, to our mutual surprise, that when his prosthetic limb was removed and I did energy manipulations in the open space where only his phantom limb existed, he could feel the presence and contact of my healing hand, and I could feel the presence of his absent limb in that same empty space. Our energy fields were truly interacting. He felt a sense of trapped energy in his stump which wanted to flow down and out his leg. He was able to facilitate this process with my energetic guidance.

However, he could find no way to let this moving energy exit his leg. He mentioned that he could not let go of the energy, of the pain, of the leg. He came to feel and to see that he had in fact not yet accepted the loss of his leg, and that his pain allowed him to hold on to his old self-image as a two-legged athletic young man. The long-deferred grief began to surface for him following this visceral realization, and a prolonged course of traditional supportive psychotherapy set the stage for him to mourn his loss, to ener-getically let go of his amputated leg, and to begin to create a new self-image and a new life.

This case graphically validated several aspects of the energy model of the human organism. The palpable presence in empty space of his physically absent but sensately painridden phantom limb illustrated the reality of the etheric level of the energy field quite vividly to both of us. Electromagnetic measurements of this phenomenon in other amputees would provide objec-tive validation. Related measurements in plants, the so-called phantom leaf phenomenon of Kirlian photography,[18] provide a striking parallel to phan-tom limb pain. For my patient, the experience of holding on to his energy allowed this rather concrete, un-psychologically minded man to bridge the gap between his body and his emotions. His physical energetic experience allowed him to recognize his emotional pain. When his emotional pain has been released, the energetic pain will also resolve. Presumably both levels of his field, the emotional body as well as the etheric body, will be cleared by this process.

Conclusion

Certainly a state of deep comfort similiar to that produced in energy healing can also be created by meditation, self-hypnosis or biofeedback, but I've found in my patients that the feeling is deeper and more profound with energy work. Not only does the feeling of comfort and safety allow talk-therapy to proceed more directly, but also there appears to be a direct healing effect on the organs of the body that is not possible in non-energy techniques. Patients can experience a part of themselves that is more than just their physical bodies or their minds at work, it is the subtle energy body.

As was mentioned in Chapter 2, alternative therapies like acupuncture and homeopathy may also work by creating and harnessing minute but measurable changes in the patient's own electromagnetic field. However, I do not think that energy healing is simply a mechanical process of interacting electrical and magnetic fields, because the key ingredient is the state of mind of the healer. Unless the healer is in a mood of compassion and altruism, the process simply does not work. So the healer must feel the emotion of acceptance and unconditional love toward the patient, not sexual love, but simply the respectful acknowledgement that the person before you is on his or her own healing path that has an inner integrity and wisdom which must be honored. If this attitude of compassion is not cultivated, true healing cannot occur. If it is cultivated, then mutually resonating energy fields can envelope both therapist and patient in a transpersonal trance that can be profoundly healing for both participants.

References

1. Montague, Ashley, *Touching: the human significance of the skin*, Harper and Row, New York, 1971.
2. Ellenberger, Henri, *The Discovery of the Unconscious*, Basic Books, New York, 1970.
3. Rama, S. and Ajaya, S., *Yoga and Psychotherapy: the evolution of consciousness*, Himalayan Institute Press, Honesdale, PA, 1976.
4. Leskowitz, Eric, Life energy and western medicine, *Advances*, Fall, 1992.
5. Lavine, L. and Grodzinsky, A., Electrical stimulation of repair of bone, *J. Bone Joint Surg. Amer.*, 69(4), 626–630,1987.
6. Burr, Harold Saxton, *Blueprint for Immortality: the electric patterns of life*, Neville Spearman, London, 1972.
7. Sheldrake, Rupert, *The Presence of the Past: morphic resonance and the habits of nature*, Time Books, New York, 1988.

8. Jung, Carl, *Man and His Symbols*, Doubleday, New York, 1964.

9. Tart, Charles, *Learning to Use Extrasensory Perception*, University of Chicago Press, Chicago, 1976.

10. Grinberg-Zylberbaum, J., Human communication and the electrophysiological activity of the brain, *Subtle Energies*, 3(1), 25–44, 1992.

11. Becker, Robert, *CrossCurrents: the perils of electropollution, the promise of electromedicine*, Tarcher, LA, 1988.

12. Ravenscroft, Trevor, *The Spear of Destiny*, S. Weiser, York Beach, ME, 1975.

13. Bailey, Alice, *Esoteric Healing: A treatise on the 7 rays*, Lucis Press, New York, 1953.

14. Brennan, Barbara, *Hands of Light*, Bantam New Age, New York, 1988.

15. Bruyere, Rosalyn, *Wheels of Light*, Fireside Books, New York, 1994.

16. Krieger, Dolores, *Accepting Your Power to Heal*, Bear and Co., Santa Fe, 1993.

17. Benor, Daniel, *Healing Research: holistic energy medicine and spirtuality*, Helix Books, Munich, 1993.

18. Gerber, Richard, *Vibrational Medicine: new choices for healing ourselves*, Bear and Co., Santa Fe, 1988.

For further study:

Rev. Rosalyn Bruyere
Healing Light Center Church
PO Box 758
Sierra Madre, CA 91025
(818) 306-2170

Barbara Brennan School of Healing
PO Box 2005
E. Hampton, NY 11937
(516) 329-0951
http://www.barbarabrennan.com

Nurse Healer's Association
P.O. Box 444
Allison Park, PA 15101-0444

chapter four

Clinical intuition and energy field resonance

John Tatum

Introduction

Although the concept of energy fields in the human body has been fundamental to Eastern thinking and medicine for centuries, it has only recently
been accepted in the West. However, awareness and interest in this area has
increased recently, with more books, studies, and seminars appearing as the
1990s come to an end. The new Office of Alternative Medicine of The
National Institute of Health has identified energy medicine as one area
worthy of study and research. More studies are needed to expand our knowledge of the role of the human energy system in health, illness, and healing.

As more clinicians become interested and knowledgeable about the
human energy field, discussions concerning integrating this knowledge into
current accepted medical practice are needed. As an allpoathic physician, in
the early years of my exposure to alternative practices utilizing the human
energy field, I was in conflict about whether to follow the accepted medical
pattern or to embrace the alternative. I now see the obvious need to respect
the knowledge and wisdom of both approaches and integrate them. In this
chapter, I will share my experiences in energy medicine, how I have integrated this into a standard psychiatry/psychotherapy practice, and how the
interaction of the energy field may explain intuition and other common
human expereinces. I'll also include some of my thoughts and experiences
in integrating energy medicine concepts in the medical setting.

I hope that by sharing some of my experiences over the past fourteen
years, readers who are not knowledgeable in the area of energy medicine
will gain more of an understanding of this area. Although it is no substitute
for research, hopefully such sharing will add to the general knowledge and
interest and will encourage scientific study. If this area is new to you, then

0-8493-2237-5/00/$0.00+$.50
© 2000 by CRC Press LLC

as you gain actual experiences, you will not only have validating experiences, but also find a feeling of familiarity. I am reminded of the quote by William James, "A new idea is first condemned as ridiculous and then dismissed as trivial, until finally, it becomes what everybody knows".[1]

Many studies outside the scope of this discussion have validated our ability to affect and read other people, animals and even things, both locally and at a distance, through our mental intention. The concept of *subtle energy* and a human energy field have been proposed as the mechanism of action to explain these phenomena. As Larry Dossey, M.D. stated at the keynote address at the Second Annual Alternative Therapies Symposium in Orlando in April, 1997, the phenomenon is real, but we still do not fully understand it. Therefore, we should use the idea of subtle energy as a metaphor. He suggests our consciousness and intention may be much more powerful than we imagined and may not need a mediating subtle energy to create its effects. Hence, I will use the term *subtle energy* as a metaphor in this discussion.

Background and body centered meditation

After medical school, I did my psychiatry residency at the Sheppard Pratt Hospital in Baltimore, Maryland because of my special interest in psychotherapy. Moses Sheppard was a Quaker who believed that psychiatric patients should be treated with dignity and respect at a time when there was still much abuse of mental patients and much misunderstanding of mental illness. Sheppard Pratt Hospital was also founded on a strong belief in psychotherapy and many of the pioneers in the field were there at one time or another.

I served the first two years after my training as a Navy psychiatrist at the Naval Training Center in Orlando, Florida. I then entered private practice in 1979 as the chief consultant to a community mental health center. I did three and a half years of weekly phone supervision with Robert Langs, M.D., a psychoanalyst in New York who has written extensively on the bipersonal field. He focuses more on the interaction between the therapist and patient and the therapist's contribution to the interaction, than traditional psychoanalysts. Implicit in his approach is the belief that the patient unconsciously knows the therapist's mind and has to address the therapist's issues before he/she can address their own issues. I submit that we often make assumptions about our intuitive ability without being able to adequately explain the mechanism and without fully contemplating the ramifications of this ability.

Through my work with Dr. Langs, I learned much about the nature of the unconscious and how the unconscious expresses itself. I began to pay more attention to the patient-therapist interaction in the therapy. However, I abandoned the psychoanalytic model of therapist neutrality because a more active approach seemed necessary for certain types of problems, especially panic disorder, phobias, posttraumatic stress disorder, and the dissociative disorders. I completed a year of training in Neuro-Linguistic Programming,

(NLP), a hypnotherapeutic technique developed by Richard Bandler and John Grinder. From the fields of linguistics and systems theory, they studied and modeled experts in the field of psychotherapy, including Milton Erickson, Virginia Satir, Carl Whitaker, Jay Haley, and others. They broke down the interventions of these gifted therapists into steps which could then be taught; in other words, they unpacked their strategies. NLP is therefore a collection of techniques and presuppositions, (i.e., the patient has all the necessary resources to accomplish any desired goal).

After the NLP training, I studied hypnosis in more depth and became active with the Florida and American Societies of Clinical Hypnosis. For a number of years I made presentations to the American Society of Clinical Hypnosis on the subject of energy field interactions. Modern hypnosis is thought of as starting with the work of Franz Anton Mesmer and his animal magnetism. As described in more detail in Chapter 2 of this book, his work resembles modern therapeutic touch and other forms of energy medicine, all of which are based on a concept of an energetic interaction. Mesmer induced an altered state by the use of Mesmeric passes, which involved passing one's hand in a downward sweeping motion near the body. James Esdaile, M.D., a British physician serving in India in the mid 1800s also used the Mesmeric passes down the body to induce patients into a trance for anesthesia prior to surgery. Interestingly, sweeping the hands up the body has a stimulating rather than calming effect.

I was first introduced to energy fields and energy centers (chakras) in 1983 by W. Brugh Joy, M.D., through experiential seminars and through his first book, *Joy's Way*.[2] Brugh graduated from medical school with honors, did his specialty training in internal medicine at John Hopkins, and a fellowship at the Mayo Clinic. He returned to the University of California and was selected as the youngest director of medical education. Once while doing a routine insurance physical examination, the thought occurred to him that since the liver is such an active organ metabolically, perhaps he could sense that with his hand. He moved his hand above the patient's body and did not feel anything over the liver, but did feel a sensation over the upper abdomen. Over the next several months, he mapped the body, doing so surreptitiously so patients would not think he was strange. After completing this project, he was amazed one day while in a bookstore to see a book on display opened to a diagram of the human energy centers, or chakras, which matched his findings. Brugh was very excited and wanted to share this with his colleagues, but not surprisingly, this information was not well received. He later developed chronic relapsing pancreatitis, which is often fatal. He left medicine, feeling his life depended on a change of vocation. After extensive travels throughout the world, he became a metaphysical teacher and one of the leaders in human energy work.

In Brugh Joy's "Foundational" seminar,[3] one learns (among other things) to scan someone's body with the hand (feeling for the warmth or tingling or vibration as it is passed over each of the major energy centers), and to balance the energy fields. The recipient of this balancing also feels warmth, tingling or vibration, and at the end usually is relaxed with a feeling of well being. Psychological breakthroughs are not uncommon.

By now there are many disciplines of energy field balancing and body energy work including Reiki, therapeutic touch, and cranio-sacral therapy. Energy awareness is a fundamental part of the work of many modern massage therapists. These scanning and balancing techniques are all based on the premise that there is an energy field about the body which is fundamental to health and sickness, and this energy field can be affected by another person's energy field. These therapeutic approaches are all therefore examples of energy field interactions between people.

My introduction to Brugh Joy affected me profoundly. The practice of medicine had become somewhat cold and mechanical to me. Brugh Joy awakened my heart and soul and reconnected me with the heart and soul of medicine and healing. This occurred through his words in the group sessions, through experiencing an energy balancing by him, through the experience of feeling another's energy field, and through the group healing ritual. I was very moved when I first scanned someone's body and felt the energy emanating from the chakras. Through this experience and a group healing ritual, I felt like I was being reintroduced to an ancient mystery that is a fundamental part of medicine and life.

My first experience with body-centered healing actually occurred at my first Brugh Joy conference in 1984. Halfway through the two week conference, the attendees were to start two and a half days of silence and fasting. I was 36 years old and had a twenty year history of a peptic or acid stomach. This was characterized by burning, pain, and a hungry feeling in my upper abdomen, which occurred if I had not eaten in several hours. I coped with this by eating often and using antacids, which I carried with me all the time. The conventional wisdom of the time was that this was due to a genetic predisposition, and indeed, my father had the same problem.

As I went into the silence and fasting, I knew I was going to have a problem with this and did not want to take antacids during the fast. It then occurred to me for the first time that there might be a psychological component to this symptom. I put on a particular t-shirt I liked, and walked in the desert. When I returned to my room, I instinctively felt I wanted to lie down, placed my hand over my upper abdomen, and started to focus deeply on that area, being open to whatever might come up. I soon got in touch with angry feelings, which eventually went back to some early childhood anger. I somehow knew that I could trust this process and that if I kept going deeper into the feelings, I would find a resolution. I therefore went with the anger, exaggerating it in my mind as I lay quietly in the bed. Soon I was wielding a sword at real and imagined adversaries. I passed through anger regarding my early life and feel I went into the archetype of anger and destructiveness, the devil. I was then suddenly catapulted out of the anger and pain into a blissful state where I experienced great peace and felt that I had unusual insight: a state of cosmic consciousness. In this state, I felt I understood good and evil and how we as humans split off both ends of the spectrum. I felt like taking a ritual shower of cleansing and renewal. While undressing, I was shocked by the t-shirt that I had felt compelled to put on at the beginning of this meditation. This had been my favorite t-shirt and I now understood why. This shirt was sky blue with a dark center circle on the front with a night scene and a reddish full moon. In the center was an owl, talons exposed, swooping in for the kill. The blue represented the calm and intellectual front I presented to the world. In the darkness of my unconscious was this repressed anger, represented by the red moon and the owl. Unconsciously, I had been showing the world my underlying issue.

I never again felt the same about the shirt, realizing how I had been acting out my repressed anger by wearing it, and I don't think I ever wore it again. I got through the fasting without difficulty and without antacids, and have not had a recurrence of the acid stomach. Occasionally, I will feel a knot in my upper abdomen, but I now know there is something I need to work on and the symptom soon resolves with the body centered meditation.

The next step in my evolutionary process was a ten day intensive Vipassana meditation retreat[4] in 1985. This was the beginning of my learning about body centered meditation, and it began a deepening of my understanding of how to work with posttraumatic stress disorder and early childhood traumas.

Vipassana meditation[5] comes from Burma and India and was reportedly handed down through the generations from the Buddha. There are different branches within this non-Tibetan Buddhism, with some differences in technique. Some involve noticing what arises in the mind and body while meditating, not reacting to it, and letting it go. Others, like the training I attended, involve continually scanning the body with a narrowly focused awareness. This focusing is done during the first three days of the ten day retreat. We were to focus merely our attention on the sensations associated with the breath at the nose. The focus at first included the whole nose, later only the ring at the opening of each nostril, and eventually a pinpoint on the ring of one nostril. During these three days, the mind gradually became steady and sharply focused. Starting on the fourth day, we were to start systematically scanning the body with this pinpoint awareness. I was immediately amazed at the intensity of the feelings as I scanned my body. I lingered at the areas of maximum pain. At times, there was an associated psychological and emotional component. It was obvious that I was getting in touch with previously repressed issues.

As a psychiatrist and psychotherapist, I felt I understood why the retreat leaders stressed continually scanning the body. By intently focusing my attention on my body, I was breaking through my previously held defenses and getting in touch with realizations and memories and with their corresponding physical and emotional components. I understood that the purpose of the scanning was to desensitize myself by degrees, to prevent flashbacks from overwhelming me with early traumatic memories or current realizations. By this time in my life, I had done enough psychotherapeutic work on myself that I was not worried that I would not be able to handle the material, so I spent much of my time focusing intently on areas of maximum discomfort. It became evident that the most intense feelings correlated with the location of the chakras or energy centers as I had learned them from Brugh Joy, (see Appendix at the end of this chapter).

In the succeeding months, I continued this type of meditation, focusing my attention on the areas of my body where I felt discomfort at a particular time. This form of meditation can also be described as a type of self hypnosis, since hypnosis is a narrowing of one's focus of attention with a resulting absorption in the area of focus and a blocking out of everything else.

At times my discomfort would simply resolve. At other times, repressed thoughts, memories, and feelings would come into awareness. The repressed material was either an awareness in the present moment, or a series of associations leading back to an early childhood trauma or misunderstanding. Once the repressed material came into consciousness, resolution of the conflict usually followed spontaneously. If the issue was from the past, then over the next few minutes and hours, there would be an automatic process whereby the mind would ascend back up the previous chain of associations, resolving those situations based on the insight gained from the core memory.

Body centered meditation and therapy

After gaining considerable personal experience over the next year with this body centered meditation, I began to ask some patients where they had feelings in their body as they talked about some problem. With their consent, I would pace them into focusing more on the discomfort and deepening it. Sometimes formal hypnosis was used and sometimes age regression, but usually I used an indirect hypnotic approach. This involved simply suggesting that the person focus their attention on the area of discomfort in their body and either face and accept it in the present or set the intention to go to the origin of the feeling.

I preferred to use this light form of hypnosis because I wanted the patient to stay in touch with the present reality and not have a flashback. A flashback is an experience in which a person relives a trauma so completely that they are in the situation in the past and lose awareness of the present reality. This can be difficult for the inexperienced therapist to handle, difficult for the patient, and can traumatize the patient again.

Adding this body centered component to the therapy was extremely helpful, and brought faster and more specific results. After adding this to my psychotherapy, I was gratified to attend an American Society of Clinical Hypnosis meeting in 1988 at which Ernest Rossi, Ph.D., demonstrated essentially the same technique. Dr. Rossi trained with Milton Erickson, the pioneer of indirect hypnosis and an important figure in the acceptance of hypnosis as a clinical tool, and has himself become a leader in clinical hypnosis. At the conference, Dr. Rossi demonstrated a technique in which he had subjects identify the body sensations associated with the issue they wanted to address. He then induced hypnosis and suggested they go more deeply into the sensations, with an eventual resolution of the presenting complaint. Rather than just focus on the feelings in the body, sometimes he would focus on urges to move the body. In one demonstration, the subject had the urge to spread his arms like an airplane. Dr. Rossi encouraged him to actually spread his arms and to deepen the feeling of being an airplane. He felt empowered, expansive, and now he felt he could overcome the temerity he was previously experiencing. This way of working is reminiscent of Frederick "Fritz" Perls, the founder of Gestalt Therapy,[6] who would also have someone "be the plane" if that image appeared in a dream.

This body centered approach ties in with psychodynamic psychotherapy. We think of transference as the transferring of feelings from the past onto the present situation. If a father was constantly critical of a patient as a child, the patient might, through the process of transference, feel the therapist making an interpretation is being unduly critical, or complain about normal feedback from the spouse as being overly critical. The most successful interpretations occur when the patient associates to the past and the therapist can then point out the pattern from the past being transferred onto the present, both in and out of the therapy. With posttraumatic stress disorder, however, interpretations alone are not sufficient. The patient must go back and remember at least a representative sample of the trauma in order for resolution to occur.[7] Often, the trauma has been repressed and therefore must be brought up into consciousness for resolution.

Whether we are dealing with a recurring maladaptive pattern, or a transference reaction stimulated by the therapy, or with an early trauma, we want to help the patient bring up into consciousness the origin of the problem. In my experience, unconscious unresolved experiences are always accompanied by feelings in the body; these feelings are almost always centered in the chakras. I had blocked these body sensations in myself until I started the body centered meditation process, and most of my patients have also done so. The sensations in the energy centers are usually experienced as tightness, burning, or pressure. It is usually easy to get a patient to tune in to these sensations. After the patient has had an opportunity to relate the problem, I simply ask, "Where do you feel this problem in your body?" Most patients are able to answer this question, though they had not previously been aware of any such body sensations. If they are not able to answer, I may ask them to close their eyes and scan their body, or notice the sensations in the body as they focus on their breath, or notice feelings in the body as they focus on the problem and their feelings about it. Focusing on the breath helps to relax the person as well as calm and steady the mind and it shifts their awareness to their body.

Energy field interaction and intuition

As I continued to work with patients in this way, I started to notice that when I asked a patient where they were having sensations in their body, I was already having corresponding sensations in my own body. When their issue was resolved and the sensations in the patient's body disappeared, the sensations in my body also appeared. Often, the sensations resolved in one energy center and then moved up to the next center in the patient, and the same process also happened with me. These experiences are consistent with the model of a human energy field - there are energy field interactions between the therapist and patient. The energy is not limited to one body, but radiates from the body and affects any other fields in the environment.

It is my hypothesis that the human energy field interaction also plays a role in clinical intuition. One definition of intuition given by Webster is "the power or faculty of attaining through direct knowledge or cognition, without rational thought or inference."

This implies that information can come into conscious awareness from the unconscious mind. Therapists talk of having frequent intuitive flashes during sessions. With some patients we know, or sense, a great deal about them from the beginning. We use our intuition to guide us regarding when to make an interpretation and how to phrase it for a particular patient. We tailor our approach to the individual, guided by our intuition. During indirect hypnosis, we somehow know just what to say to facilitate the process. With the nonverbal dissociated patient, I usually am able to sense what they are dealing with and what interpretation is needed to help them resolve the current crisis.

Certainly we use our experience and training as well as our knowledge of the patient as we evaluate a situation. We use such objective signals as the patient's words, demeanor, voice characteristics, and body language. However, if these were sufficient, would we need the term *intuition*? Intuition implies that our unconscious mind accesses information from some other source than the five physical senses. The human energy field model would offer an easy explanatory model: intuition is a resonance between interacting energy fields.

The next step in my training helped me deepen my understanding of energy field interaction, the chakras, and the unique states of consciousness associated with each chakra. In 1988, I was a participant in the Nine Gates Mystery School.[8] I later served as a staff member for several years. This twenty day program is led by Gay Luce, Ph.D., a transpersonal psychologist, and author of hundreds of articles and five books. She has been a writer for and consultant to the National Institute of Mental Health, and was on President Kennedy's Scientific Advisory Committee. She was a three time recipient of the American Psychological Association Award for journalism.

At the Nine Gates Mystery School, we were exposed to various mystery traditions, including Celtic, Taoist, Buddhist, Sufi, early Egyptian and Greek, Native American, and Christian. The concept of a human energy field is fundamental to native traditions and was taught in ancient mystery schools. In one Tantric Yoga exercise we did at Nine Gates, one member of each pair would activate a chakra in his own body (by imagery and intent) and his partner would try to guess which chakra had been energized by noticing the corresponding activation in his own body. Participants did not find this

exercise difficult, and the assumption was that this identification was possible because of an energy field interaction. My hypothesis is that this phenomenon occurs anytime we are in rapport with someone and certain unconscious associations are triggered. Some thoughts filter up into consciousness,
resulting in an intuitive thought. The analogy of resonant tuning forks
described by Leskowitz in Chapter 3 of this book is apropos.

What I am describing here is the same as the phrase "picking up the
vibes," which was so common in the 1960s. Although that terminology is
not often used today, the concept still prevails. We are used to placing
considerable trust in our impressions and feeling of a person even though
we are not able to fully explain why we feel the way we do. This energy
field interaction and our ability to unconsciously read people would also
explain familiar experiences such as intuitively picking out compatible people at large gatherings, love at first sight, the alcoholic or adult child of an
alcoholic picking a similar person out of a crowd, and the victim of childhood
abuse unconsciously picking someone who will abuse them. I believe we
are all psychic but those who make a living at it are more gifted or more
practiced at using it for positive growth. Certainly my ability to read someone accurately has improved as I have increased my belief in the possibility.

Some therapists may wonder why they have difficulty reading patients
in this way. It was only after 2 to 3 years of doing body centered meditation
that I noticed I could also sense others using my kinesthetic orientation.
Some people, like Jack Schwarz,[9] Rosalyn Bruyere,[10] and Barbara Brennan,[11]
are evidently very visual in their mental processing because they report
reading unconscious patterns in people by seeing energy fields. Presumably
there are people who can discern the human energy field auditorily or
through other sensory modalities.

Energy field interaction in psychotherapy

I am suggesting that in the psychotherapy setting, there is an energy field
interaction which can be deepened and utilized to aid in the therapeutic
process. I have described intuition being one by-product of this energy field
interaction. The energy field interaction is also very useful in assessing and
monitoring a patient. In the psychodynamic psychotherapy that I practice,
the patient is encouraged to talk about what comes to mind and what they
have the most feeling about. If a patient is clearly over-reacting to some
current life situation, that suggests to me that an unconscious unresolved
issue is present. After the patient has had an opportunity to state the problem,
I will ask them where they are having a corresponding feeling in their body,
and silently correlate that with what I am feeling in my body. This process
would be more complicated and less accurate if I was reacting to something
outside the session or reacting in a personalized manner to the patient's
material. With the patient's permission, I will then suggest that he close his
eyes and focus on the sensations in the body. The patient will be encouraged
to either face and accept the feeling in the present or to go more deeply into

the feeling with the intention of getting to the core issue. As I sit in silence following the above directions, it is extremely helpful to be able to monitor what is going on with the patient through my own sensations. With this knowledge, checked periodically with the patient, I can intervene more quickly and more appropriately; I thus have access to more insight into the issues at hand.

The sensations in the body will remain unchanged, deepen, resolve completely, or resolve in one energy center but then move up to another. If the tightness remains, I continue to work on this, and if it is the end of the session, I give some suggestions about how the patient can continue to work on this on their own. If the tightness in the body intensifies, I know that the patient is going more deeply into the issue. And if the tightness resolves, the patient feels better and usually has new insight.

When the discomfort is resolved in one chakra, the energy may move up to the next and activate it with a corresponding good feeling. On the other hand, if there is discomfort at the higher chakra, then that becomes the new focus. As the therapy progresses, session to session, the patient gradually works through the unconscious unresolved issues. The energy naturally moves up the body and activates the upper chakras. There will be many cycles through the body, with the energy activating progressively higher chakras. As the therapy progresses, it changes from a focus on illness to a focus on growth and development.

The growth phase is also greatly facilitated by the therapist's ability to monitor where the patient is energetically focused. This monitoring is particularly important when working with the upper chakras because this spritual domain may be completely new territory to the patient who may have no experience with the issues involved with the upper energy centers, how they feel in the body, or how to work with growth in those areas.

When dealing with the upper chakras, the person may not have a complaint for the session because they are not dealing with a problem which disturbs them. My approach is still the same and that is to have the person tune into the feelings in their body. If, for example, the patient complains of a headache and I feel activity on top of my head, I would suspect they are dealing with a seventh chakra issue (transcendance, universality, etc.) rather than just having a headache. Headaches are common when working with the seventh or crown chakra. This is because the person is in a lower state of consciousness but their natural growth and development is trying to bring them into a higher state of consciousness.[12] Since this concept is new to many patients, they may not realize what is happening, and their current life may not currently support this higher state. Hypnotically pacing them into this seventh chakra state will usually not only release the pain, but bring them into a new level of awareness. This same approach is also used with any chakra the patient had not been able to activate in a positive way.

Being able to monitor the energy field interaction is also extremely helpful in assessing the patient's strengths or gifts. Helping a patient to know

where they are gifted, and helping them to develop their gifts, is an important part of the pyschotherapeutic process. I can receive hints as to where a
person is gifted by how they affect me energetically. When a person first
comes into treatment with a history of childhood abuse, I would normally
expect them to have considerable blockage in the third chakra (located in
the upper abdomen) and also the second chakra (in the pelvic area) if there
is a sexual component. But if working with such a patient, I notice sensations
in my lower chest or fourth chakra, then I hypothesize that the patient is
gifted in the heart center with the ability to feel compassion (see Appendix).
On the other hand, if I frequently notice feelings at the top of my head, the
patient is probably gifted spiritually. The shared feelings of tightness or even
pain mean the patient's energy is still blocked, but frequent activity there
usually indicates that the patient has strengths in that area which will manifest after the blocks are resolved. In other words, they are trying to activate
this chakra, but the block in the lower chakra is limiting the available energy
and thus preventing full expression of these strengths. Jack Schwarz dis-
cusses this same phenomenon from his visual perception of the energy fields
in *Human Energy Systems*.[13]

Energy field interaction, psychotherapy, and active energy work

Up until this point, I have focused on the feelings I pick up from the patient.
But if their body is radiating this life force energy and it is impacting my
body, then I must also be affecting them, even if they are not aware of it
consciousnsly. It seems very important to me then to make sure that I am
calm, centered, and not blocked myself. By "centered," I mean being in the
state of awareness associated with the heart chakra. According to Brugh Joy
and others, this energy center is associated with unconditional love, compassion, healing, and being in touch with the innate harmony of the universe.[14] I think it is also associated with acceptance of the reality of what is.
I believe that in order to resolve something, we need to face and accept the
reality of the situation, and our feelings about it. This means being in the
heart state of consciousness as we face the situation. Patients usually do not
have their heart activated when they are struggling with a problem. I am
feeling the uncomfortable sensations in my body that correspond to their
discomfort, but I am also activating my heart, which they in turn pick up,
helping them to heal.

I believe that this is what a mother does when she comforts her child.
For example, an Italian study examining the use of pain medications with
hospitalized children found (to the experimenter's surprise) that a visit by
the mother reduced the child's pain more than any of the pain medications,
including narcotics. Similarly, when my patients accept my role as energetically supporting them, their therapy seems to be more effective. My patients
will frequently say that they are able to resolve issues, focus on their heart

center, and relax or meditate during the therapy session more easily than when at home, even if the work done in the session is done in silence.

In my earlier therapy work, I was satisfied to be with the patient in their pain, staying centered as described above. But after doing some work in 1995 with Anamika, a graduate of Barbara Brennan's School of Healing,[11] I learned that I could play a more active role in helping release a patient's energy blocks while still maintaining my therapeutic stance and distance. This is done mainly through intention, but also through projecting energy with the palms or fingers. There is a saying, "Energy follows intention." This means that if you set an intention to project energy, then energy does in fact get projected. This phenomenon is well known not only to healers, but also to martial artists. If you think about it, there are many things we do by setting an intention, without really knowing how we actually do it. For example, we do not understand the details of how we walk, raise our arm or talk, much less how we can tell ourselves to wake up at a certain time, raise our skin temperature, or lower our sweat gland activity. We can see the results of those activities, though, and we can subjectively feel a difference when we do set an intention to project his human energy. In my 10 years of Aikido treaining and teaching, we practiced at each session projecting this energy and this was fundamental to the effectiveness of the art. In tests of strength, an experienced Aikido practitioner could easily overpower a physically larger but energetically inexperienced person. Projecting the energy by intent was necesssary to accomplish this result.

I have also had training in EMDR (Eye Movement Desensitization and Reprocessing),[15] and I will often use that technique to clear some issue and its corresponding energy block. My energetic monitoring of the patient's progress and my energetic support is a helpful addition to the basic EMDR protocol. I believe that EMDR in fact works by disrupting energy field patterns induced by trauma, and my energetic support facilitates that process.

In my clinical practice, I also teach my patients how to work energetically with themselves, outside of the sessions. The fifth step of the Body Centered Meditation that I teach[16] involves first centering the heart, then noticing where there is a feeling or block in the body, and then resolving it by facing the feelings in the present or going back to the source of the problem. The therapist must know a patient well and know that they will not be thrown into a traumatic memory if he recommends that they trace something back to the past. Through my work with Anamika, I have learned that I can sometimes instruct patients to resolve something by simply setting an intention to clear the energy block in the body. This clearing is also done in various hands on energy healing systems, but can also be accomplished with the mind alone, by thinking of the painful sensations as negative energy to clear from the body. You may imagine sweeping motions, with the energy moving down the body and out the feet, with positive energy coming into the body through the crown, root, or abdomen. You may also imagine just expelling the negative energy or use some other metaphor for the clearing.

Anamika believes in the importance of the patient's asking for help from the spiritual realms, and with time I have gained more confidence that such transpersonal help is available. See Chapter 13 of this book for a discussion of the types of information that have been accessed by this approach. This request by the patient also helps him or her enter a more surrendered state of mind which also facilitates the healing process. This surrender is similar to the step taken by Alcoholics Anonymous, in acknowledging a higher power. The role of spirituality in healing is being taken more seriously by many well respected authorities as the gap between science and spirituality is bridged.

Energy field interactions in the medical setting

The following vignette illustrates the power of energetic interactions.

I was called as a consultant to assess the agitation of a hospitalized elderly man who was dying of cancer. I was surprised when I reviewed the chart and saw the patient because he had been in a deep coma for several days. The patient did appear quite agitated, and his breathing was very labored. The patient was unresponsive to my speaking to him, but I felt he might on some level be frightened of his approaching death. I placed one hand over his heart chakra, and the other over mine. I then set the intention to help induce him into a heart centered, unconditionally accepting state. When centered at the heart, one can accept death as a natural phenomenon. One is in tune with the way the universe works, rather than being frightened and trying to fight the inevitable.

The patient became very calm within a few minutes, and his breathing became normal. After removing my hand, he remained in a peaceful state. He died peacefully in the early morning hours. I had given him no medication, my only interaction being energetic.

I think it is extremely important for physicians and health care workers to be open to the idea of energetic interactions. Patients frequently complain that the modern physician is well-versed in technical matters, but is not comforting and has a poor bedside manner. Modern medicine has certainly stressed the technical aspects, but has not stressed the power of the inter-personal relationship. Simply stated, the physician or health care worker needs only to realize that there is an energetic interaction involved in their work. They can help their patients by setting their intention to project heal-ing, compassion, care, and acceptance of the situation. There can also be physical touch, but it is not necessary. This caring approach can be extremely comforting and helpful to the patient, and can greatly increase the health care worker's joy in work. I think many physicians are unhappy because they started practicing medicine to become helpful healers but ended up becoming technicians instead. Also, as Larry Dossey notes in *Healing Words*,[17] the physician's attitude has been shown in double blind experiments to have a therapeutic effect in the medical setting.

Conclusions

I encourage readers to be aware of the energy field interactions in their private and professional life, and to realize their associated responsibility to set the intention to have a positive influence on others, rather than to be indifferent or to have a negative influence. Bringing more awareness into energy field interactions will greatly enhance the power of the interactions. Setting the intention to extend this positive energy will result in very positive reactions from people. Awareness of energy field interactions will also help us to be humble and honest, since our patients and others are also reading our fields, and are thus able to know our inner truths, at least on an unconscious level.

I also encourage the reader to appreciate and respect the value of professional training and the professional relationship with its associated boundaries. Although hands on healing is a powerful modality, one can maintain a professional stance and still do energetic healing, as described here. The reference list is a good place to start for someone interested in learning more about this subject. Most importantly, though, experiment and discover for yourself what the role of energy fields is in your own life.

Appendix

> Seventh Chakra: at the top of the head, associated with the spiritual.
> Sixth Chakra: at the forehead; associated with vision, insight intuition and thinking.
> Fifth Chakra: at the throat; associated with speaking one's truth and living that truth.
> High Heart Chakra: at the upper mid chest; associated with joy.
> Fourth (Heart) Chakra: at the lower mid chest; associated with unconditional love, compassion, caring, healing, harmony, and acceptance.
> Third Chakra: at the upper abdomen: associated with the sense of self, with power, fear, anger, and the need to control.
> Second Chakra: at the pelvic area, below the navel and above the pubic bone; associated with the sexual.
> First Chakra: at the perineum; associated with survival and our connection with the earth.

References

1. James, William, in *Light Emerging*, Brennan, Barbara Ann, Ed., Bantam Books, New York, 1993.
2. Joy, W. Brugh, M.D., *Joy's Way: a map for the transformational journey*, J. Tarcher, Los Angeles, 1979.
3. Brugh Joy, Inc., www.brughjoy.com.
4. Vipassana Meditation, www.dhamma.org/.
5. Hart, William, *The Art of Living – Vipassana Meditation*, Harper and Row, San Francisco, 1987.

6. Perls, Frederick, *Gestalt Therapy Verbatim*, Bantam, New York, 1969.

7. Putnam, Frank, *Diagnosis and Treatment of Multiple Personality Disorder*, Guilford Press, New York, 235, 1989.

8. Nine Gates Mystery School, www.ninegates.com.

9. Schwarz, Jack, www.mcn.org/b/aletheia.

10. Bruyere, Rosalyn, *Wheels of Light: a study of the chakras*, Simon & Schuster, New York, 1990.

11. Brennan, Barbara Ann, *Hands of Light*, Bantam, New York, 1988.

12. Keyes, Ken, *Handbook to Higher Consciousness*, 5th ed. , Living Love Publishers, Coos Bay, OR, 1975.

13. Schwarz, Jack, *Human Energy Systems*, Dutton, New York, 1980.

14. Joy, Brugh, *Avalanche: heretical reflections on the dark and the light*, Ballantine Books, New York, 140, 1990.

15. Shapiro, Francine, *Eye Movement Desensitization and Reprocessing: basic protocols, principles and procedures*, Guilford Press, New York, 1995.

16. Tatum, John, *Body Centered Meditation*, unpublished report.

17. Dossey, Larry, *Healing Words*, Harper, New York, 1993.

For further training:

Vipassana Meditation: http://www.dhamma.org.

Nine Gates Mystery School: http://www.ninegates.com.

Brugh Joy, MD: http://www.brughjoy.com.

Barbara Brennan School of Healing
PO Box 2005
East Hampton, NY
(516) 329-0951
http://www.barbarabrennan.com

chapter five

Hypnosis, yoga, and psychotherapy

Susana A. Hassan-Schwarz Galle,

> The human experience is an experiment in movement and thought and form. The most that we can do is comment on the movement, the thought and the form, but those comments are of great value if they can help people to learn to move gracefully, to think clearly, to form — like artists — the matter of their lives.[1]

Background

One experiment in movement, thought, and form is psychotherapy, a change-oriented process which includes a therapist and a client (patient) in "a contractual, empowering and empathic professional relationship."[2] In the evolution of Western psychotherapies, the experiential ones expanded the focus of the "talking cure," psychodynamic or behavioral, directive or client-centered, to getting "in touch" with feelings lodged in the body (e.g., Perls, Reich, Lowen). They thus laid the basis of body-mind work.

Transpersonal (Jung, Grof) and humanistic (Maslow) approaches went beyond conflict resolution, relief from suffering and insight (Freud), towards higher development of the self. Erickson's hypnotherapy[3] paved the way for a psychobiological approach to mind-body healing.[4,5] Thus naturalistic approaches to hypnosis utilize the client's resources, strengths, and rhythms as a springboard for therapeutic interventions. In recent decades, the increasing East-West dialogue has propelled holistic views, fueled by the surge of spirituality, and by scientific discoveries linking the brain, emotions, and behavior. Body, mind, and spirit converge as one reality in the psychotherapeutic experience.

This chapter presents hypnosis and Hatha yoga as transpersonal methods that work synergistically in psychotherapy.* Matter and energy are
equally considered. Hypnosis accesses state-dependent learning, becoming
a vehicle for symptom removal and conflict resolution. Once hypnotic communication reaches the subconscious mind, it modifies emotions, physiology,
and cognition.[6] Reframing and future orientation are invaluable tools for the
renewal of beliefs, attitudes, and behaviors. Yoga postures (Asanas) and
breath control (Pranayama) reshape the flow of subtle energies organized as
chakras which regulate the bodymind.**

Hypnotic suggestions for inner focusing and the meditative essence of
yoga, entail attention training and mindfulness.*** Relaxation is a by-product
of both. While hypnosis works through verbal and sensory images (visual,
auditory, kinesthetic) influencing body-mind processes, Hatha yoga also
involves various body movements. Of particular interest is Astanga yoga as
taught by Sri K. Patabhi Jois[7] because its poses are linked to form a heat-
producing, "movement breathing system" (scientific Vinyasa). Moreover, the
Astanga form uniquely emphasizes breath control (ujjiah pranayama), locks
(bandhas), and proper gaze (drsti), making it a prime energy modality.****
The ancient Astanga yoga, retrieved from the "Yoga Korunta" and revised
by Patabhi Jois, was used over a thousand years ago for various ailments.
The Sun Salutations were said to relieve depression and anxiety. The name
of the Astanga primary series, "Yoga Cikitsa," means "Yoga Therapy." Kripalu yoga is another relevant approach, which sequentially balances willful
practice and surrender. This form also encourages the selective use of breathing techniques and locks during the poses. Its spontaneous posture flow
becomes a "meditation in motion," facilitating emotional and spiritual integration.***** In yoga therapy, the added energy balancing that emanates from
the therapist enhances self-awareness and induces changes. Examples of
therapist-induced energy balancing include adjustments and assists during
the yoga poses, hands on healing, polarity therapy, and coordinated breathing with the client.

* Ha-Tha = Sun-Moon, male-female polarities united or harmonized through yoga.
** Chakra (Sanskrit) = vortex of energy. The chakras are seven centers of vital energy and
consciousness. Each center corresponds roughly to an anatomical area and a major gland in the
human body. Yoga psychology and medicine take into account each center's physiological,
psychological, and metaphysical attributes to asses imbalances and design corrective treatments.
For details see C.W. Leadbeater, (1987). The Chakras, Ill.: The Theosophical Publishing House,
and Rama S. et al, (1977). Yoga and Psychotherapy, Honesdale, PA.: Himalayan Institute Press.
*** Meditation (from Sanskrit) = medha-tation, getting to the wisdom within.
**** Ujjiah (Sanskrit) = victorious breath. Ujjiah entails breathing through the nose and feeling
the breath from the throat, which produces a hissing sound that enhances energy and engages
the mind. The bandhas are contractile movements (chin, abdomen, and perineal) which
modulate the flow of vital energy (Prana) in the chakras, and turn it into spiritual energy.
Varying "gaze" or drsti (nine looking places) for different poses helps focus attention and
direct energy flow. For details see L. Schultz & J. Gates, (1996). Astanga Yoga: A Practice
Guide, Nauli Land Press, S.Fco., and Freeman, R., (1993). Astanga Yoga: The Primary Series,
Boulder: Delphi Productions.
***** See Desai A., (1985). Kripalu Yoga: Book II, Lenox: Kripalu Publications.

Both hypnosis and yoga had their own trajectory as separate treatment modalities since ancient times.[8] Currently, hypnotherapy includes traditional, authoritarian approaches and forms emphasizing inner direction.[9,10,11] Hypnosis steadily gained acceptance in medicine and psychotherapy. Cheek's[12] ideomotor questioning was widely applied here, as an open-ended method designed to elicit nonbiased responses from the client's subconscious mind. Yoga is also making headway into the medical field. Various studies affirm its usefulness for improving physical well-being, reducing anxiety, and enhancing personality.[13,14] Yoga outcomes were translated into psycho-physiological variables, ranging from blood pressure to objective indexes of anxiety, but they vaguely referred to changes in the patients' energy state.

Assessing an individual's energy system before and after yoga and hypnosis can enrich our understanding of how these methods affect physiology. Some authors[15,16,17,18] addressed the human energy fields directly in relation to illness and health, as well as the role of consciousness in the dynamics of healing. Leskowitz'[19] "psychoendocrine" model of hypnotizability introduced an energy "link" in hypnosis, by connecting pituitary function, the third-eye chakra, and the eye-roll technique of assessing hypnotizability.[20]

The author's case studies illustrate the alliance of hypnosis and yoga therapy in exploring a client's deep conflicts and facilitating inner awakening. Yoga and hypnosis connect body and mind through breathwork, relaxation, images, and memories. In addition, yoga is like an open window overlooking an individual's energy field, since the body actively moves in it. The physical body reveals one's history and present status, in addition to bearing the marks of fatigue, sadness, anger, tension, fear, pain, distractibility, etc. Initially, the therapist's body reading[21] and later on, the Body Scan meditation, give therapist and client entry into the client's psyche, regardless of any verbal communication.* Eloquently put in the Baghavad Gita[22] Sloka[7] is this holographic model of body-mind-spirit:

> Look at my body, Arjuna. You will see the entire universe there — all that moves and all that [seems to be] moving, as well as anything else you wish to see. And all are part of the same, which is me.

Theoretical considerations

As a matter of interest and inquiry for those who practice psychotherapy, one may ask, when does trancework end and yoga therapy begin? Or is this combination better labeled "yogic trancework," a trance of self-balancing and integration?

---

* Body Scan meditation = mindful (internal) observation of one's body, part by part, while doing ujjiah breathing.

Hypnosis is a state-dependent phenomenon occurring in all forms of life. In humans, it has survival value and is based on the mind's capacity for dissociation. D.B. Cheek noted that hypnotic states are characterized by literal understanding, access to imprints from stressful or traumatic experiences, inhibition of physical activity, diminished verbalization, decreased need for food and metabolic rate, increased tolerance for pain and resistance to infection, and homeostasis. Attention is turned inward, fixated, and one is more receptive to suggestion. Wolinsky[23] suggested that Deep Trance phenomena create and maintain symptoms, and that the "therapeutic trance" is comparable to the "no-trance state" in which a person's perceptions flow freely during meditation. Thus it is simpler to use the symptomatic trances to heal rather than inducing new trances. Hypnosis in a therapeutic context is a valuable method for self-discovery and mobilizing one's healing powers, moving from illusory beliefs to a reality orientation.

How does one walk the thin line between a therapeutic trance and meditation? We may need to redefine the new hypnotherapies as covering a spectrum of consciousness ranging from reverie to relaxed, alert awareness. Psycho-biologically, hypnotherapy healing can be viewed as a process which involves the normalization of ultradian rhythms. Werntz's[24] research attested to the role of the hypothalamus in regulating ultradian rhythms, in cerebral dominance, nasal dominance, and autonomous nervous system integration. In Chapter 6 of this book, Osowicz described her clinical experience with yogic breath and ultradian hypnosis in relation to hemispheric dominance. These authors' contributions and this writer's own work support a connection between the psychophysiology of states of consciousness and Yoga, a link between neuroscience and Eastern healing.

Biofeedback technology already makes it possible to assess subjective states during psychotherapy, by giving precise signals about physiological responses that accompany particular emotions and ideas. Peper et al.[25] described biofeedback as potentially opening holistic and transpersonal horizons. Green et al.[26] used EEG feedback to look at brain wave patterns and their control in experienced yogis. One reason for studying yoga masters through the magnified glass of science is the assumption that they have reached the highest level of inner balance, control, and integration. Although nature is constantly in motion, the yogin(i) can tame the fluctuations within, through an assiduous psycho-physical practice known as a Patanjali's Astanga (eight limb) Yoga.

Yogic "stillness" (Nirodha), far from mere catalepsy or trance, is a state of readiness in which consciousness opens up to new modes of experience. This mindedness becomes a point of contact between Hatha yoga and hypnotic trancework. The emphasis is on wakefulness, acute awareness and feelings of reality. For the psychotherapy patient, yoga poses, breathing, and meditation become tools for removing distractions, awakening consciousness, and reaching the transcendental self, the healer within. In the Yoga Sutras[27]

> Pain, depression, tremor of the limbs, [wrong] inhala-
> tion and exhalation are accompanying [symptoms] of
> the distractions. For this reason, a 'qualified teacher'
> must guide the yogin (1.31).

And further:

> The projection of friendliness, compassion, gladness,
> and equanimity toward objects — [be they] joyful, sor-
> rowful, meritorious or demeritorious — [bring about]
> the pacification of consciousness. (1.33)

In meditation practice, those four virtues are radiated to everyone. Translated into a psychotherapeutic stance, this means acceptance and nonjudg-
ment, accompanying, guiding, reflecting the client's inner search, and watch-
ing lovingly his or her transformation. This points out the importance of the
quality of the therapist's consciousness and therapist-client communication
in each therapeutic encounter. The author's own experience highlights the
invaluable potential of the above stance through the dance and whirlwinds
of psychotherapy.

Clinical uses

In hypnosis- and yoga-assisted psychotherapy, questions recommended for
the initial meeting include:

1. What is (are) the main problem(s) or complaint(s) or symptom(s)?
2. How does the client communicate through words and body language
   (self-presentation, body reading, energy patterns)?
3. What prior interventions have there been (treatment or self-help)?
4. What is (are) the client's goal(s) in therapy (direction)?
5. Personal and family history, significant others, facts, and accomplish-
   ments (identity, identifications, key events/trauma).
6. How to reach (via empathic dialogue) the client's resources to open
   up resolution paths (utilization).
7. Empowering the client to access inner wisdom, and to become the
   agent of growth (from victim to architect of the self).
8. What are the client's and therapist's mutual impressions (percep-
   tions/expectations)?
9. Is the client receptive to spirituality (helpful but not necessary)?

Most people are not used to paying close attention to their subtle energy
"goings-on." Instead, they live in their minds. Hence, in this therapy clients
may refer back to their first transformational experiences as "magic." What
seems to be mesmerizing for some is the emotional release that comes from
mental and body work, combined with spiritual integration. As the chakras

open up, a changed energy flow modifies physiological responses and breeds new perceptions in place of old problems. Some clients perceive hypnotic trance as the path to internal changes while others awaken their energy by holding yoga postures and breathing — hence, the nexus between "matter" or "body-mind matters" and "energy." Yoga therapy here entailed a combination of poses, breathing, and meditation in the context of therapeutic dialogue. The metaphysical and historical aspects of yoga poses have been outlined elsewhere.[28,29,30]

The following case summaries convey how this therapy works in an individualized way, creating viable alternatives to other failed methods. There will be a detailed discussion about one woman who completed psychotherapy three years ago. At yearly follow-ups, she reported satisfaction with her life as well as being symptom-free. Vignettes from another two closed cases, a man and a woman, illustrate breakthroughs in the process. All clients experienced significant shifts in self-awareness and lifestyle.

Case Illustrations of Hypnosis- and Yoga-Assisted Therapy

All three individuals selected had unsuccessfully tried conventional approaches, including extensive medical work-ups, medications and/or other forms of psychotherapy.* The first woman reported here sought help with chronic headaches. She also wanted to lose her excess weight in preparation for pregnancy. Secondly, a man came in feeling despondent on the eve of turning fifty. Thirdly, there was a woman whose lack of concentration and depression were linked to post-traumatic stress disorder (PTSD).

Hypnosis was applied diagnostically and generated therapeutic changes. Using ideomotor signals, motivational factors surrounding the symptoms, their origins, and subconscious resistances to get well were explored. Once the stresses or traumas were re-experienced and released in a trance state, reframing and future orientation enabled these clients to create their own solutions and "see" them projected onto the screen of the mind's eye. They were all talented hypnotic subjects (registering 3 to 4, on Spiegel's eye-roll technique) who learned self-hypnosis, and practiced it as needed. In every case, body reading revealed energy congestion around the head and neck, as well as bodily constriction related to each client's symptoms. Yogic breathing and poses induced relaxation and changed awareness.

The first patient, Mary, also joined a small yoga therapy group which offered postures, breathing, higher self meditation, weekly journaling, and the individualized use of imagery and affirmations. The middle-aged man, Joe, had extensive yoga therapy to deal with negative body image and physical pains prior to hypnotherapy. The woman with PTSD, Claire, had been sexually abused by her father, and mistrusted human connections. Through yoga therapy she felt sufficiently free and empowered to accept hypnotic suggestions.

* The real identity of all patients reported was disguised to protect confidentiality.

Case 1: Mary

Mary was 37 years old, married ten years, and parenting a 4 year-old son. Her husband, age 39, was a chemist. She worked part-time in the health field. Her mother, stepmother, and mother-in-law, all lived out-of-town. Her father died tragically in a car accident shortly before her son's birth. She had a brother, two years younger, and a half-brother (a teenager) from the father's second marriage. In childhood she endured much instability, with recurrent moves due to the father's job changes. She had friends but was often separated from them. An overachiever in school, Mary enjoyed science and sports. As a teenage athlete, her running team competed nationally. She went through puberty at age 13, just when her parents got divorced, and she became sexually precocious.

Engaged at age 18, she broke up with her fiancee at her parents' insistence. In college, Mary became sedentary, felt lonely, and empty. Overeating led her to gain excess weight, which she lost through Weight Watchers. In graduate school she met her husband and married him two years later. She converted to his religion, which initially displeased her father, a minister. The relationship with her mother was strained by her mother's demands and rigid discipline, in contrast with her father's warmth and ease. Two years prior to therapy, Mary had a miscarriage, which left her insecure about having any more children. During the course of psychotherapy, she got pregnant, as planned, and gave birth to her second son at full term.

Mary had 20 individual sessions, the first 13 of which entailed primarily hypnotic exploration. Then she had 5 lengthy sessions of yoga therapy combined with hypnosis. The last 2 sessions consisted of hypnosis in preparation for labor and delivery along with resting yoga poses for late pregnancy.[31] She attended 10 sessions of a yoga therapy group, until her pregnancy necessitated individual work. She initially sought help for chronic headaches and obesity. Since some of her headaches manifested two or three days prior to menstruation, she received a hormonal diagnosis. With acupuncture and analgesics she obtained partial relief. She was also diagnosed as having reactive airways, and just prior to this therapy she received steroid treatments for asthmatic wheezing.

During our initial telephone contact, Mary sounded vulnerable yet eager to work on herself. In person, she presented as calm, short, with a large body-build, broad shoulders and a big chest, having well-developed muscles from her athletic days. Her face was round and young-looking, with an intent expression and a winning smile. Her voice was animated. Her breathing, quick and shallow, reflected tension. In the first session, she learned about hypnosis. Under ideomotor questioning, her finger signals indicated that her inner mind accepted hypnosis as a means to understanding her symptoms and solving problems. She also decided to change her diet, eliminating refined sugar and wheat. Mary's contact was warm and personable. She expressed positive expectations for our work.

The second session brought out her long-standing separation anxiety through hypnotic age-regression back to birth (birth imprint). Born six weeks early, Mary endured her mother's problems with labor contractions. Both parents were happy and relieved after the delivery of the tiny baby. Since age five, she had fears of being abandoned because of the parents' fights and their frequent uprooting. At puberty, her parents' divorce left her angry but she would not release it for fear of losing control. In the ensuing years she got headaches, the worst one during her mother's visit following the birth of her son. Mary realized the meaning of her headaches in relation to contained anger. Through hypnosis, she learned to modulate the intensity of her pains, and to stop hurting altogether. Into the future she visualized herself pain-free. By the third session, she had no more pain.

For two sessions after that, hypnosis was used to explore Mary's weight. With her new diet she had lost six pounds, but was medically advised to lose some more prior to conceiving. In college, overeating assuaged her loneliness and homesickness. Being overweight protected Mary against care-free sexuality. Meeting her husband genuinely filled the emptiness. She redefined her experience as one of loneliness, more than depression. Through future orientation she projected herself as a "pretty fit" mother.

In the sixth session, trancework gave Mary access to the unresolved attachment to her late father. She felt angry because of his untimely death just before she became a mother. She visualized a "last conversation" with him, in which the father expressed his happiness about her having a baby. She also forgave him for his first, negative reaction to her husband and for other mistakes. She also "saw" herself hugging him while he uttered the good-bye she had missed. To complete her griefwork, Mary acknowledged on a higher level (meditative), his legacy to her: creativity, perseverance, and a good sense of humor.

By the seventh session, she remained headache free and lost 12 pounds. Her weight loss continued. For the next few sessions, her focus shifted to the relationship with her mother and mother-in-law. The fear of hurting their feelings, kept her angry inside. Mary now viewed herself as more sensitive to her own feelings and needs. Rather than holding everything in, she imagined herself freeing up. A one-time recurrence of her headache during her mother-in-law's visit led to feeling the pent-up anger in her chest, saying, "Let me out." This experiential work relieved her pain, and made her feel lucky to have someone (the therapist) attuned to her feelings. Amidst these internal changes, she and her family moved to a larger home, which she handled effectively. After their vacation, Mary discovered she was pregnant. She quickly controlled her low blood sugar headaches from early pregnancy, and scheduled more rest in order to deal with early evening fatigue.

On the fourteenth session, yoga therapy began with a Body Scan meditation which deepened Mary's awareness of herself and the proprioceptive changes of pregnancy. While she lay down, comfortably propped in the Fish pose, an open-ended journey of inner exploration a la Phoenix Rising (see Reference 30) was suggested to her. Mary's eyes filled with tears concerning her desire to hold on to the pregnancy, to give it new impetus, and she again relived the loss stemming from her parents' divorce. The Fish pose, usually eliciting matters of the heart by opening up the chest in a supported upper-back supine position, also allowed Mary to release residual feelings about her miscarriage. After that, a Chakra Meditation (including all seven centers) along with energy balancing facilitated Mary's integration of her thoughts and her more primitive feelings, the heart and the womb. This laid the ground for bonding with her unborn baby, through nurturing and protective color visualizations. For example, Mary had spontaneous images of peach-colored energy spreading in the womb. She was also given a home program of warm-ups and modified yoga poses for each trimester of pregnancy.* The seventeenth session, yoga therapy was organized around the following assisted poses: Bridge, Child, Spinal Twist, Corpse. Abreaction during the Child pose stimulated further trancework as this pose once again evoked chaos around her parents' divorce. She put these memories in a new per-spective by affirming her own wisdom and experience as an adult, which enabled her to care for the frightened thirteen year-old she once was. She felt calm and self-confident at the end.

The last two sessions, one month before giving birth, Mary came in to prepare for labor and delivery. In the nineteenth session, utilizing her preferred imagery, a script was collaboratively created for her to try out. The last session, her feedback about what worked, led to a final version taped for Mary's use until the delivery. Suggestions were added for post-partum wellness and trust in the body's wisdom. Trance induction entailed the metaphor of a flower opening out, blossoming, emphasizing the visual properties, texture, and natural fragrance. A summary of labor and birth rehearsal ensues:**

1. going in and out of trance
2. relaxing abdomen and back
3. distributing blood evenly throughout the body
4. beginning contractions only when the baby is ready to come out
5. feeling the baby moving into the proper position inside the womb
6. dilation of the cervix, enabling the baby to come out comfortably, head down

---

* The energy impact of moola bandha, or the root chakra lock in yoga practice, is very relevant here. Moola bandha, which involves contraction of the perineal body by lifting the pelvic floor and doing ujjiah breath, also resembles the Kegel exercises indicated for pregnancy. This "root" movement (at the first energy center) ignites the fire within and brings things into life.

** The author gratefully acknowledges the late David B. Cheek, M.D., mentor and friend, for his assistance as an experienced obstetrician and hypnotherapist.

7. as dilation occurs and the baby travels down the birth canal, strengthening the abdominal and perineal muscles to push and relax as needed

8. relaxing and allowing everything to be open, letting all muscles be as open as needed

9. feeling contact with the baby coming out, feel it like a gentle, stroking sensation

10. visualization of a healthy baby placed on her lap for breastfeeding

11. welcoming the baby into this world

12. feelings of fulfillment, unconditional love for the newborn, hugging the baby, being separate and being one

Mary's son was born in the middle of the night at home. He was delivered by her son's coach, a family friend (luckily a midwife!) while Mary's midwife was en route. Mary experienced his birth as wonderfully satisfying and pain-free, a great improvement on her first son's birth. Using self-hypnosis, she had listened to the labor and delivery tape regularly as well as doing prenatal yoga. She was ready and confident. She was given illustrated materials with instructions to practice postpartum yoga and meditation.

On follow up, Mary stated that many things were resolved within her. Hypnosis helped her with physical symptoms and to explore conflicts. She practices self-hypnosis at times of stress or whenever she does not get enough sleep and needs re-energizing. She no longer has headaches. Her efforts at completely losing the weight gained during pregnancy include self-hypnosis, having set a date to achieve her weight goals within two years of giving birth. For added support with a sensible diet she went to Weight Watchers. She does yoga and Tai Chi, which she views as physical and spiritual conditioners. Mary's lifestyle changes, benefiting her whole family, also reflect shifts in self-image and awareness, particularly her ongoing interest in self-help and listening to her own needs along with her caring for others.

In summary, psychotherapy with Mary addressed three major matters:

1. grief (the parents' divorce, the father's sudden and tragic death, the miscarriage)

2. new habit development and reinforcement (diet, weight control, relaxation, breath)

3. preparation for labor and delivery

The headaches were closely tied to her emotions, e.g., anger and grief. Once these emotions were released and integrated, little remained to be done symptomatically. In this instance, energy work with hypnosis and yoga were clearly combined to deal with internal blocks. Changes in consciousness enabled Mary to transcend her symptoms, resolve long-standing problems, and develop in her words, "a new orientation to life", integrating the methods she learned in psychotherapy.

Case 2: Joe

Joe began therapy at age 49, amidst a severely depressive episode. He also complained of upper back pain, colitis, and hypochondriasis. For over a year, he had been unsuccessfully treated with acupuncture and holistic medicine. He also took minor tranquilizers. Joe was an investment manager, happily married, with two married children and two grandchildren. His body posture suggested a heavy burden on his shoulders. He seemed tightly put together. His breathing was shallow and uneven. He spoke in a monotone and battled tears. Strongly verbal, he derived moderate relief from recounting his sorrows. Recent dreams of "winding roads" and "dark tunnels with no clear exit," helped him to tune into his experience of uncertainty, lack of direction, fears of being trapped, and losing control.

Feeling heard and understood by me was crucial to Joe's engagement in psychotherapy. But he dramatically reconnected with his deep feelings in two yoga therapy sessions. In one session, the Body Scan meditation made Joe sharply attend to the tight knots within, and he noticed how his mind and bodily sensations were connected. In another yoga therapy session, the assisted Camel pose produced an exhilarating new sense of power and freedom. In this pose, the client kneeled against the wall and facing it. He bent backwards in a chest opening movement and breathed fully, while he was firmly backed up by the therapist sitting behind with her feet supporting Joe's nape and upper back along the spine. Through this energy exchange, he suspended his habitual fearful pose and experienced the capacity to project himself creatively and positively onto the future.

Hypnosis was introduced later on for handling residual pains, and for deeper exploration of his fears. Pain control happened easily within one session. Subsequently, he practiced on his own with periodic reinforcement in our sessions. In observing his panics attacks and indecisiveness, Joe tied them to the early admonitions of his overprotective mother and the lack of an active paternal influence. As he released the fears, higher self meditation affirmed his own perceptions and actions. Joe increasingly valued whatever came from within, relying less on expert opinions. His posture straightened up and his facial expression was brightened by a smile. His outlook shifted from early retirement to planning for a second vocation, and cultivating new interests with his wife. He took up yoga and balanced his diet. He began facing life with directness, at work and at home. As his growth process gained momentum, Joe worked on himself independently, taking long breaks from our sessions. His increased self confidence and sense of competence led to termination after three years of psychotherapy. On follow up, he reported continued enthusiasm and confident handling of crises.

Case 3: Claire

Claire was 38 years old, single, and an artist. Her parents had divorced when she was an adolescent, after her mother learned of the father's sexual abuse.

Claire looked drained, having problems with memory and concentration. Her facial expression reflected fear but her speech was flat and intellectual, as though she were talking about someone else (dissociation). She began psychotherapy after the break up with her live-in boyfriend, expecting that antidepressants would "do the trick." She had adverse reactions until finding the right medication for her.

Initially mistrustful of hypnosis, she was open to energy work through yoga since her body felt tense and achy. While doing ujjiah breathing, she went through a Body Scan and assisted yoga poses. The sequence of Mountain, Child, and Corpse poses was selected to elicit grounding, self-nurturance, and relaxation, respectively. Claire spontaneously visualized colors, "like floating in the galaxy." She had an intense "rush" which made her body feel "truly alive" for the first time in years. With this awareness came surges of energy in Claire's daily life, improved concentration and memory, as well as optimism.

In subsequent sessions, she opened up to hypnotic exploration. For the first time ever, she connected with the intense feelings about sexual abuse by her father and released them as she abreacted. Up to then, her memories of the traumatic events were devoid of affect. She also retrieved her self-image as "a confident kid" prior to the abuse, and radiated self-confidence forward into the future, by using her own color imagery of "warm gold." Further on, she made spiritual contact with a most beloved family member, her deceased maternal grandmother, feeling her presence and protection within. Silent tears rolled down her face. Claire's transformation began. She made new friends, became more productive at work, and set up goals. She also decided to decrease and stop the antidepressants. She enjoyed yoga, which brought out many memories and a new awareness of herself and her family. Changes in her posture included opening up her chest, smoothing her humped back, and breathing fully. She became more expressive and her voice sounded animated.

Claire went on vacation for one and a half month, and came back with renewed enthusiasm about working on herself and with me. She was developing a trusting alliance, and handled her "down" times without despairing. During the therapist's vacation she got depressed again and, upon psychiatric consultation, she resumed taking medication, which calmed her down but also made her "seal off" from inner exploration. This fact added to financial constraints, led Claire to stop our sessions. But the seeds planted in seven months of therapy were not lost. For a while, Claire called periodically, and further on wrote me about her progress. The last I heard she was to relocate because of a fine job offer.

A note on the turning point in each case

The turning point in each of these cases can be schematically put as follows: Mary "watched" her emptiness following the family break up during adolescence, and the anger about being bereft of a home. In "feeling free" from his energy knots, Joe discovered his reservoir of strengths and took decisive steps on his own. Claire sensed a "rush" flowing up her body once she freed up energies trapped to mask the trauma that deeply scarred her. These experiences entailed key changes in energy and consciousness. In hypnosis, these clients recreated their inner reality. Yoga therapy helped create awareness of a changing energy flow in their body-mind along with increased mastery.

The individual reports as to what made a strong impression upon each of them, all reflected a higher order learning beyond learning about their problems. Bateson's notion of "deuterolearning" (1942) comes to mind. As the body-mind behaved differently through the hypnotic and yoga experiences, these clients developed new ways of looking at themselves and the world. They thus released outdated premises. These individuals were encouraged to go inside, draw from their inner source (the higher self, inner teacher), affirming their movement towards growth. My own experience entailed a gradual shift from teacher and guide to that of being a witness of their unfolding.

Closing remarks

Questions remain about the differences between hypnotic trances and yogic trances:

1. What is the psychobiology of healing in therapeutic hypnosis and Hatha yoga?
2. Do they belong to related fields of meaning and healing?[32]
3. What is their precise connection with the phenomena which we call *attention*?

As attention and relaxation change consciousness, they modify the energetic flow in the body-mind. In psychophysiologic language, energy changes are reflected in breath, heart rate, and brainwave patterns, etc. For example, EEG tracing during deep hypnotic states resembles those of stages III and IV sleep. The author's experiments with brainwave monitoring during her own yoga breathing practices showed selective increases in alpha during ujjiah, and a balancing of alpha and beta during anuloma viloma (a form of alternate nostril breathing). In contrast, the hypnagogic state induced by a colleague's suggestion to daydream produced some high amplitude theta waves.* Into the future, advances in brainwave mapping may help discriminate between the EEG spectrum found in hypnotic states and yoga. This information could be utilized to train individuals who are poor hypnotic subjects to enhance the natural capacity for trance. Thus, biofeedback technology may become a tool for the scientific study of consciousness and

---

* These observations were made during an individualized workshop on EEG biofeedback with psycho-biologist Joel Lubar, Ph.D., at Southeastern Neurofeedback Institute.

energy in relation to psychophysiology. One could learn more about how breathing affects brain blood flow, which in turn modifies brainwaves, muscle tension, etc., along with thought patterns. We could then see greater convergence among the findings on energy fields, neuroscience, and the art of psychotherapy.

At this state of the art, the author's clinical experience indicated that this holistic approach works deeply and effectively as a catalyst for the client's inner healing. Its transpersonal aspect is essential because utilizing altered states therapeutically opens up information channels not accessible to ordinary consciousness. Hypnosis and Hatha yoga are, respectively, a more mental or more physical way of probing into the subconscious realm. In tandem, these two methods can substantially impact mind and body. The states of profound absorption associated with yoga and hypnosis enhance creativity. Hence, these states of consciousness hold good potential for re-patterning old perceptions once the stressful or traumatic imprints are recognized and released.

Whether one emphasizes therapeutic hypnosis or yoga therapy at different stages in psychotherapy depends on the clients' needs and inclinations, as shown in these case summaries. Both methods are conducive to learning relaxation, focusing attention, and adopting an observer or "witness" stance vis a vis one's experience. Moreover, hypnosis and yoga discourage rationalization. Hatha yoga is a fine system of personal ecology, known to strengthen, rejuvenate, and heal. One may attain comparable results from other energy-based disciplines such as Tai Chi or Chi Gong. The author chose Astanga and Kripalu yoga as deeply transformational forms, whose ways of working with energy benefit those tending to somaticize distress, or weakened by chronic conditions, as well as those who are fit. But true psychotherapeutic effects manifest when yoga goes with shifts in consciousness which carry over to daily attitudes and behavior.

Interestingly, with all the clients described here, presenting symptoms took up a minor portion of therapy. For they became deeply involved in self-discovery. All clients made positive lifestyle changes as well. The therapist's interventions as guide and empathic witness, together with energy work, mirrored the clients' receptivity to growth. Their improved attention, relatedness, self-esteem, productivity, and well-being were linked to greater awareness, flexibility, and clarity of perception. The essence of these clients' spiritual transformation is cast in poetic verse from Kahlil Gibran:

> And a man said, Speak to us of Self-Knowledge.
> And he answered, saying ...
> Say not, "I have found the truth," but
> rather, "I have found a truth."
> Say not, "I have found the path of the soul."
> Say rather, "I have met the soul walking
> upon my path."

For the soul walks upon all paths.
The soul walks not upon a line, neither
does it grow like a reed.
The soul unfolds itself, like a lotus of
countless petals.[33]

References

1. Zukav, G., *The Seat of the Soul,* Simon & Schuster, New York, 1989.
2. J.K., Zeig, and Munion, W.M., Eds., *What Is Psychotherapy? Contemporary Perspectives,* Jossey-Bass, San Francisco, 1990.
3. Erickson, M.H., *Innovative Hypnotherapy: the collected papers of Milton H.Erikson on Hypnosis,* Vol. IV, E.L. Rossi, Ed., Irvington, New York, 1980.
4. Rossi, E., *The Psychobiology of Mind-Body Healing: new concepts of therapeutic hypnosis,* W.W. Norton, New York, 1986.
5. Rossi, E. and Cheek, D.B., *Mind Body Therapy: methods of ideodynamic healing in hypnosis,* W.W. Norton, New York, 1988.
6. Brown, P., *The Hypnotic Brain: hypnotherapy and social communication,* Yale University Press, New Haven, 1991.
7. Barte Nhi, *Yoga et Psychiatrie: Reflexions a Propos d'une Technique Ancienne de Recherche de la Liberation,* Tete de Feuilles, Paris, 1972.
8. Miele, L., Astanga Yoga, *International Federation of Astanga Yoga Centers,* Rome, 1994.
9. Frankel, F., Significant developments in medical hypnosis during the past 25 years, *Int. J. of Clin. & Exper. Hypnosis,* 35, 231–247, 1987.
10. Spiegel, H. and Spiegel, D., *Trance and Treatment: clinical uses of hypnosis,* Basic Books, New York, 1978.
11. Gilian, S., *Therapeutic Trances: the cooperation principle in Ericksonian hypnotherapy,* Brunner/Mazel, New York, 1987.
12. Cheek, D.B., *Hypnosis: the application of ideomotor techniques,* Allyn & Bacon, New York, 1994.
13. Arpita, Physiological and psychological effects of Hatha Yoga: a review of the literature, *J. Int. Assoc. Yoga Therapists,* Vol. 1, No. I & II, 1–28, 1990.
14. Patel, C., Yoga-Based Therapy, in *Principles and Practice of Stress Management,* Lehrer P. & Woolfolk, R., Eds., 2nd Ed., Guilford, New York, 89–13, 1993.
15. Gerber, R., *Vibrational Medicine: new choices for healing ourselves,* Bear & Co., New Mexico, 1988.
16. Karagulla, S. and van Gelder Kunz, D., *The Chakras and The Human Energy Fields,* Theosophical Publishing House, Illinois, 1989.
17. Shealy, N. and Myss, C., *The Creation of Health: merging traditional medicine and intuitive diagnosis,* Stillpoint, Walpole, NH, 1988.
18. Brennan, B.A., *Hands of Light: a guide to healing through the human energy field,* Bantam, New York, 1987.
19. Leskowitz, E., The Third Eye: a psychoendocrine model of hypnotizability, *Amer. J. Clin. Hyp.,* 30:3, 209–215, 1988.
20. Spiegel, H., The Hypnotic Induction Profile (HIP): a review of its development, *Ann. New York Acad. Sci.,* 296, 129–142, 1977.

21. Dychtwald, K., *Bodymind*, J.P. Tarcher, Los Angeles, 1977.
22. Sri Swami Satchidananda, *The Living Gita: the complete Bhagavad Gita and commentary*, Henry Holt, New York, 1988.
23. Wolinsky, S., *Trances People Live: healing approaches in quantum psychology*, Bramble, Norfolk, CT., 1991.
24. Werntz, D., Bickford, R., Bloom, F., and Shannahoff, S., Alternating cerebral hemispheric activity and lateralization of autonomic nervous function, *Human Neurobiol.*, 2, 39-43, 1983.
25. Peper, E., Ancoli, S., and Quinn, M., Eds., Mind/Body Integration: essential readings in Biofeedback, Plenum Press, New York, 1979.
26. Green, E.E., Green, A.M., and Walters, E.D., Biofeedback for Mind/Body Self-Regulation: Healing, and Creativity, In Peper et al., Eds., *Mind/Body Integration: Essential Readings in Biofeedback*, Plenum, New York, 125–140, 1979.
27. Feuerstein, G., *The Yoga Sutras of Patanjali: A New Translation and Commentary*, Inner Traditions, Vermont, 1989.
28. B.K.S. Iyengar, *Light on Yoga*, Revised Ed., Schocken Books, New York, 1977.
29. Swami Sivananda Radha, *Hatha Yoga: The Hidden Language*, Shambala, Boston, 1987.
30. Lee, M. and Reynolds, N., *Phoenix Rising Yoga Therapy*: training manual, Housatonic, MA, Phoenix Rising, 1992.
31. Jordan, Sandra, *Yoga for Pregnancy*, St. Martin's, New York, 1987.
32. Whitmont, E.C., Form and Information, *Noetic Sciences Review*, (31), 11–18, 1994.
33. Gibran, K., *The Prophet*, Knopf, New York, 1983.

For further study:

Susan Galle, Ph.D.
Body-Mind Center
1325 18th St., NW, Suite 212
Washington, D.C. 20036
(202) 429-9552

International Association for Yoga Therapy
c/o Dr. George Feurstein
P.O. Box 1386
Lower Lake, CA 95457
(707) 928-9898
Fax: (707) 928-4738

chapter six

Yogic breathwork and ultradian hypnosis

Darlene A. Osowiec

Ancient scriptures of Swara Yoga (the Yoga Science of Breath), an important component of Ayurvedic medicine, described the various patternings of air flow and their relationship to physiological, psychological, and personality states.[21] Swara Yoga taught the importance of pranayama, breathing exercises which balance the patterns of inspiration and expiration, thereby regulating the autonomic nervous system.[6] The yogis described the nasal cycle, the regular alternation in nasal congestion from one nostril to another, in intimate detail, and they emphasized that by being aware of one's own breathing and thereby consciously controlling one's state of consciousness, the individual can prevent disease. Until quite recently, little attention was given in the West to the wisdom of Eastern theories of philosophy and psychology. This chapter examines relationships between yoga breathing techniques and outcomes with a naturalistic approach to hypnosis first introduced by Milton Erickson, M.D. The connection between hypnosis and ultradian rhythms, postulated by Ernest Rossi, Ph.D., is also explored.

Yogic breathwork, consciousness, and the transpersonal

Four major components are usually involved in the practice of yoga:

- physical postures/asanas
- relaxation
- meditation
- breath control[2]

0-8493-2237-5/00/$0.00+$.50
© 2000 by CRC Press LLC

Arpita reports that studies involving yoga have shown relief from anxiety, hypertension, and psychosomatic disorders by controlling voluntary and involuntary nervous functions. Western medicine and psychology have been looking to these ancient disciplines for such practical purposes as symptom relief. Yet, what is the larger purpose of these heretofore esoteric practices? A discussion of consciousness and its transformation is in order.

In the early part of this century, William James wrote in 1935 of other types of consciousness beyond the ordinary, saying that our ordinary consciousness:

> ...is but one special type of consciousness, whilst all about it, parted from it by the filmiest of screens, there lie potential forms of consciousness entirely different. We may go through life without suspecting their existence; but apply the requisite stimulus, and at a touch they are all there in all their completeness, definite types of mentality which probably somewhere have their field of application and adaptation. No account of the universe in its totality can be final which leaves these other forms of consciousness quite disregarded.[12]

It is here that we have a notion of the *transpersonal* — that which is beyond our normal waking state of consciousness, our culturally and socially imposed sense of who we are, our ego or personality.

In yet another definition, the phrase "altered states of consciousness" simply means basically different (from ordinary consciousness) without implying better than or worse than.[25] It is here that we can draw a commonality between yogic breathwork and meditation, for example, and hypnosis. Both techniques allow the individual to access altered states of consciousness and both can tap into a transpersonal dimension. As a result, the individual moves beyond experiencing himself or herself as a fixed entity; instead, he or she is opened to experience oneself as a fluid process capable of transformation. The ancient yogic study of the breath is a vast and intricate science which maps the relationships between breathing rhythms and states of consciousness.[20] Yogis have long been known to consciously control their autonomic nervous systems. They mapped the flow of prana (life energy) through introspective experiments. Swara yogis, focusing on the science of the breath, specified and codified intricate correlations between psychological states and the way the breath was flowing. A rhythmic cycle of the breath is a necessary component for an individual's balance.[20] Yogis considered nostril breathing and air flow to be so important that they properly attuned their breathing before undertaking any particular activity.

Ajaya[1] writes that Swami Vivikananda likened the breath to the flywheel of a machine. The flywheel carries the motion to finer and finer parts until ever more subtle parts of the machine are in motion. The breath supplies and regulates the motive power in every aspect of the body. "If the motion of the flywheel is not regulated, the motion of the entire machine is disturbed.

The breath affects more than the body, for the rhythms of the body, in turn, affect one's emotional and mental life."[1] The relationships between the breath and the body are reciprocal.[19]

According to yoga science, stress is an autonomic imbalance. When the balance or harmony between the sympathetic nervous system (regulating excitation) and the parasympathetic nervous system (regulating inhibition) is disturbed, stress results.[16] Proper diaphragmatic breathing, instead of the usual adult pattern of thoracic breathing is a critical mediating factor in the regulation of stress. Developing and maintaining new habits of correct diaphragmatic breathing have been shown to entirely rid the person of anxiety states.[16]

Swara Yoga emphasizes that a jerky breath produces anxiety, and the jerkier the breath, the greater the disruption to the autonomic nervous system. Our mental and emotional states affect how we breathe, and our breathing patterns are intimately related to our emotional and physical states. Breathing patterns which are habitually arrhythmic lead to habitual stress, imbalanced autonomic functioning. Further, emotional states seem to be related to an overdominance of either right or left nostril breathing. Yogic texts report that a natural and healthy condition is exhibited by the rhythmic alternation of air flow between one nostril and the other throughout the day. The continued closure of one nostril with air flowing through the other for longer than a few hours, is considered a harbinger of disease. If after six or eight hours the air flow stays continually on one side, illness is considered to be on its way. If the condition lasts for a day or longer, the situation is said to be grave.[3] As Rama et al.[21] state: "If it is true that the right side [of the body] activates a whole set of psychological and physiological functions and the left side brings into play a different set, then it would certainly be valuable to have access to an awareness of which nostril is flowing at any given moment."

While Western science views the breath in terms of oxygen intake, yoga science views oxygen intake as a minor consideration. Rather, consciousness pervades the universe. Consciousness is not simply a by-product of the physical workings of the brain. Prana, or life energy, is inhaled with the breath. Ancient manuals of yoga anatomy record at least 72,000 nadis/energy channels (some texts describe many more); these nadis are major energy pathways (subtle counterparts of the nerve impulses) coursing throughout the entire physical body. Currents of prana, the vital energy of the universe, flow through the nadis, thereby energizing and sustaining all parts of the body. The three nadis of greatest importance are called ida, pingala, and sushumna. All of these three nadis have their point of origin at the base of the spine. The ida and pingala nadis travel upward, crisscrossing each other along the spinal column, with terminating points in the left and the right nostrils respectively. The sushumna nadi travels straight upward along the spinal column and terminates at the Brahmarandra (i.e., the ventricular cavity/ the crown of the head). In the average human being, the sushumna nadi is blocked at the base of the spine, and prana flows, instead, through the ida and the pingala.[19]

Breathing which is balanced between left and right nostrils serves to devitalize the two nadis or channels, the ida (which flows through the left nostril) and the pingala (which flows through the right nostril), opening up the sushumna nadi (that which is centrally located and runs along the spinal column). Once the sushumna nadi is opened up and guided properly, "the yogi achieves liberation from all miseries and bondage. He thus merges his individual soul, or atman, with the cosmic soul, or Brahman."[19] The yoga attains samadhi, the highest stage of Yoga.[11] This is Cosmic Consciousness. Although a rare occurrence, this achievement does inform us of our human potentials and of the farthest reaches of human nature. Bucke[5] describes this evolved consciousness in people from Eastern and Western traditions.

Alternate nostril breathing (Nadi Shodhanam) is a detailed breathing practice which restores coordination between the right and the left sides of the body and brings "back into awareness a dimension of existence which has been forgotten."[21] Life energy or Prana enters the body through the breath by way of the nose. It is said that "the nose is the door to the brain and to consciousness."[14] Bhatnagar[4] notes that if an individual makes the observation of one's breath into a personal science, she or he will begin to easily notice that there is a change in the nature of consciousness according to which nostril is dominant at any particular moment.

The study of the breath and practices such as alternate nostril breathing is a movement out of the confines of consensus reality and our restrictive definitions which accept as "real" only that which is material, externally observable phenomena. Tart[25] proposes the creation of "state-specific" sciences to deal with these paradigm clashes. Often, breathing practices and meditation are used for stress management purposes and symptom relief, and the larger picture (i.e., the capacity to regulate our psychological states and levels of consciousness leading to a transformation of consciousness) is not addressed. In many ways, consensus reality is continually reinforced. As individuals become increasingly evolved in consciousness, will our social milieu and reality change? Consensus reality would necessarily change, Ferguson[8] explains, since individual transformation has collective implications.

From an Eastern perspective, human beings are more than their physical bodies. There are three "bodies," the physical body, the mental body, and the energy body, all interacting at nodal points, or centers, of consciousness. These energy centers, or chakras, (wheels of energy) are subtle bodies corresponding to various points along the spinal cord; they are associated with different states of consciousness. Chakras are the junctions of the ida, pingala, and sushumna, traveling along the spinal column. They originate at the base of the spine and terminate at the crown of the head. The reader can refer to Chapter 3 on subtle anatomy by Leskowitz in this book for further discussion.

Various practices instruct the aspirant how to achieve these higher levels of consciousness. Through properly meditating on each chakra, the individual attains a new level of integration. Polarities at each of the chakras can be integrated and synthesized, resulting in new characteristics of functioning. For example, where formerly an active/passive (pingala/ida of the sixth chakra) polarity operated, integration brings an opening to intuitive knowledge, clarity of mind, and inner vision. The process of integration at each successive chakra can be a lifetime endeavor. It is best to find a reputable teacher when one embarks on yoga breathing and meditative practices. This is a psycho-spiritual discipline of much subtlety and complexity. It is interesting to note that although this is specifically an Eastern tradition, breathing practices were also developed in Western traditions.

Western findings, hypnosis, and ultradian rhythms

There is a growing body of Western scientific evidence verifying the detailed introspective studies in Eastern yogic texts. All of human and animal life is characterized by cyclical activities with alternating periods of activity and inactivity. These cyclical occurrences are known as biological rhythms. The field of chronobiology is the general term for the area of science that examines and quantifies the mechanisms of biological time structures.[10] Behavioral chronobiology, or chronopsychology, is based on observations that, for example, animal and human task performance, motivation to do work, moods, fatigue, arousal, and sleep follow predictable patterns of increasing and decreasing efficiency.[15]

There are three categories of rhythmic activity: infradian, circadian, and ultradian. The most commonly known rhythm is the circadian rhythm which literally means "about a day." These are biological variations occurring with a frequency of 1 cycle per approximately 24 plus or minus 4 hours. Waking-sleeping, general activity, and body temperature are a few examples. Infradian rhythms are those with periods longer than 28 hours; they include circaseptan, circatrigintan, and circannual rhythms. A person's lifetime is an infradian rhythm.

Rhythms having a frequency greater than 1 cycle per 20 hours are known as ultradian rhythms, "ultra" plus "dies," higher than or beyond a day. A growing body of research suggests that the human adult exhibits approximately 90 to 120 minute cycles in physiological, neurophysiological, endocrine, and psychological and behavioral functioning. Nathanial Kleitman first discovered this 90 to 120 minute cycle from his research on sleep and dreaming. He also made systematic observations of changes in human physiology and behavior of such areas as temperature, alertness, performance, and rest. He called this rhythm that occurs throughout the day and nighttime hours the Basic Rest-Activity Cycle or BRAC.[13] Franz Halberg coined the term *ultradian* to refer to these short-term rhythms having periodicities much shorter than 24 hours. Some examples are mobility and eating, drinking, hormonal secretion, respiration, cyclicity of verbal and spatial task ability, "wakeful" fantasy, shifts in hemispheric dominance, and shifts in nasal dominance.

A groundbreaking study was carried out by Werntz[26] and Werntz, Bickford, Bloom, and Shannahoff-Khalsa.[27] Werntz[26] investigated the relationships between shifts in nasal dominance (measured with thermistors) and shifts in hemispheric dominance. She found that a direct relationship exists; that is, when the right nostril was dominant, the left cerebral hemisphere was dominant, and when the left nostril was dominant, the right cerebral was dominant. Werntz[26] defined an interrelationship between cerebral hemispheric dominance and peripheral autonomic nervous function. Her study served to establish that the nasal cycle is a "window" to, or a clear indicator of, autonomic nervous function and cerebral hemispheric activity. Werntz[26] and Werntz et al.[27] verified, in the laboratory, an ancient tenet of yoga science.

Werntz, Bickford, and Shannahoff-Khalsa[28] demonstrated in the laboratory, with forced nostril breathing, that the participants were not only able to change nostril dominance, but were also able to shift cerebral dominance to the opposite hemisphere. The researchers found that consciously-induced changes in air flow change the location of activity in the highest brain centers. What was once thought in Western science to be beyond conscious regulation (i.e., the autonomic nervous system), was now shown to be accessible to the naive human participant without the necessity of mechanical equipment such as biofeedback. These findings correspond with my previous discussion of Swara Yoga and Alternate Nostril Breathing.

Rhythmic disruptions, stress, and psychophysiological disorder

Observations and research findings from both clinical and experimental settings have pointed to the possibility that certain psychological and psychophysiological disorders involve a desynchrony in biological rhythms. Friedman[9] conceptualized a desynchronization model which states that a desynchrony in ultradian rhythms is the precondition (i.e., causal) to an outbreak of psychosomatic illness. He observed that when participants whose ultradian oscillations were being recorded became tense or stressed, their cycles not only became irregular but also became shorter in duration. Friedman proposed that control of this desynchrony should promote improvement or remission of a reversible psychosomatic illness. An extensive review of the literature on the nasal cycle, cerebral hemispheric laterality, and psychopathology can be found in Osowiec.[17]

Separate lines of research from Friedman,[9] Erickson, and Rossi[7] and Rossi[22] observed what Erickson termed "the common everyday trance" in their work with patients. Rossi[22] observed that Erickson utilized the naturally occurring shifts from right to left and left to right hemispheric functioning (an ultradian cycle) in facilitating the induction of a hypnotic trance. Rossi further observed that Erickson did this by taking note of every minute shift and fluctuation in his patient's manner (e.g., respiration, body posture, body pulsations, eyeblink, etc.); at the right moment, he utilized the patient's shift to parasympathetic ("quieting down," passive, "ida") functioning to induce trance. From his years of learning from and collaborating with Erickson as well as from observations in his own clinical practice, Rossi[22] proposed an ultradian theory of hypnosis and healing. Briefly stated:

1. "the source of psychosomatic reactions is in stress-induced distortions of the normal periodicity of ultradian cycles"
2. "the naturalistic approach to hypnotherapy facilitates healing by permitting a normalization of these ultradian processes."[22]

Parasympathetic functioning ("quieting down") corresponds to left nostril breathing, a more receptive mode of being. Rossi[23] proposes this time as an opportune moment to access the unconscious for creative problem-solving as well as for normalizing the ultradian cycles, much like alternate nostril breathing balances the left/ida and right/pingala. Remember, according to Swara Yoga, a balance between right and left nostril breathing devitalizes the ida and pingala and opens up the sushumna, accessing intuitive knowledge, unfettered by our five physical senses. Without the usual hypnotic suggestions and utilizing the patient's naturally occurring ultradian cycles, Rossi facilitates the patient's own accessing of his or her own unconscious. According to Rossi, ultradian rhythms are themselves one of the long sought psychophysiological substrates of hypnotic phenomena.

Rossi[24] describes various methods of determining which nostril is open; A simple way for the reader to assess which nostril is active at the present time is to take the index and middle fingers and gently close off the left nostril while inhaling and then exhaling through the right nostril. If there is no stuffiness, wheeziness, or noise, the right nostril is open. You can then switch and apply the same procedure to the right nostril. It is possible to experience both nostrils as being open, this indicates a switchover to the opposite nostril (try again after a few moments). When both nostrils are open for a prolonged amount of time, this corresponds to a meditative state.

In my own research,[17] I found that a person's level of self-actualization (i.e., psychological health) significantly correlates with the regularity or irregularity of the nasal cycle, an ultradian rhythm. People with greater levels of psychological health exhibit more regular nasal cycles, while people with lower levels of psychological health exhibit more irregular cycles. Self-actualization/psychological health was negatively correlated with trait anxiety, state anxiety, depression, stress symptoms, cognitive stress,and physical stress. Non-self-actualizers exhibited mostly high or moderate levels of trait anxiety and stress-related symptoms and normal, moderate, or high levels of depression.

Having demonstrated a relationship between psychological health and regularity in nasal cycles,[17] I conducted a 12 week follow up study, a case study design with five participants.[18] These five individuals also participated in the 1992 study, so these participants served as their own controls. I sought to answer the following questions:

- can daily self-hypnosis, using Rossi's[23] ultradian approach to self-hypnosis, serve to regulate a person's ultradian rhythms (i.e., the nasal cycle)?
- will changes occur in levels of self-actualization, anxiety, depression, and stress symptoms?

After instructing the participants how to record their baseline nasal cycles (recording which nostril is open every half hour throughout the day) and administering a psychological test battery, I then proceeded to instruct the participants, individually, in the practice of ultradian self-hypnosis. I stipulated that they practice the self-hypnosis, preferably twice a day, 20 minutes in the morning and 20 minutes in the evening, going into the hypnosis when they were aware that they were breathing out of the left nostril (parasympathetic, right hemispheric functioning). They recorded any insights gained during each self-hypnosis session in their nasal recording diaries. The instructions followed Rossi's[23] protocol.

The participants recorded their nasal cycles daily, at pretreatment, and at weeks 4, 6 to 8, and 12. A battery of psychological tests were administered at pretreatment and at the end of each of the time segments. The psychological tests were Shostrum's Personal Orientation Inventory (POI), Spielberger's State-Trait Anxiety Scale, Form-Y (STAI-Y), the Beck Depression Inventory (BDI), and Smith's Stress Test (ST). The Hypnotic Induction Profile (HIP), a measure of hypnotic susceptibility, was administered at the end of the study. They practiced self-hypnosis two times per day for 12 weeks.

Results showed that participants' nasal cycles became more regular with the practice of ultradian self-hypnosis. Regularity was calculated according to the operational definitions of the nasal cycle in Osowiec.[17] In brief, regularity refers to time spent breathing through each nostril during the alternating pattern of right-to-left or left-to-right shifts. Regular (i.e., Equal or Near-Equal) breathing was defined as 50 percent right and 50 percent left flow (+/− 2 percent, e.g., 48 percent right, 52 percent left). Imbalance refers to a greater than 2 percentage of time spent breathing through one nostil (i.e., 90 percent left nostril, 0 percent right nostril, and 10 percent both congested illustrates a left nostril dominance over the course of the recording period (i.e., an imbalanced cycle).

The most pronounced change occurred in participants scoring at the high end of hypnotizability, with virtually no change in those participants at the low end of the hypnotizability scale. While self-actualization (a more enduring characteristic) remained stable, participants exhibited varying degrees of reduction in anxiety and depression as well as in cognitive, emotional, and physical stress symptoms.

Clinical applications

I will highlight two cases in particular. Participant two was a 52 year-old secretary, divorced, and the mother of 2 young adults. She scored in the normal range on the POI, low trait anxiety, moderate state anxiety, low stress symptoms, normal on the BDI, and high on hypnotizability. Her main goal was to lose weight. She had been in Overeaters Anonymous for many years, but did not experience success in weight reduction. She also posed questions, during her self-hypnosis sessions, concerning the health of family members. Her nasal cycle recordings showed an unusually high percentage of both nostrils totally open compared to the other participants. That is, in 51 percent of the recording time, both nostrils were open. This both nostrils totally open pattern usually occurs as only a brief switching point between right and left nostril breathing, and this case was the only one to show this predominance. To date, I have not studied experienced meditators who would be predicted to show more of this both open pattern.

In reviewing the diary comments of participant two, I found that one specific week was the week when her stepfather was to undergo open heart surgery. When I spoke with her, this event was uppermost in her mind, along with her mother's symptoms of faintness and pains in the left arm and chest. Participant two was also dealing with a long-time emotional rift in relations among various family members.

When I spoke with her in the debriefing session, I asked her to elaborate on what she was experiencing at the time and how she coped. She assuredly replied:

> I felt that it was pretty much in God's hands. I was in Overeaters Anonymous some time ago where I learned to say the Serenity Prayer. So, I prayed the Serenity Prayer and turned it over to God. I knew there was nothing I could do to control or to change the circumstances; it's in God's hands and I felt more at peace.

According to yogic breathing practices, when both nostrils are totally open for a prolonged period of time, the individual is in a meditative state. Perhaps the prayers and the self-hypnosis sessions facilitated this meditative experiencing.

At 12 weeks, participant two had lost 10 pounds. While both scores on the POI and the BDI remained the same (i.e., normal), her state anxiety dropped one category from Moderate to Low state anxiety, and her physical stress symptoms dropped off markedly. One year later, I followed up, and she had already lost an additional 8 pounds, maintaining an ideal weight for her frame.

Her diary notes showed a process-oriented, gradual discovery of the origins of her weight problem. At the one-year post study follow up, she reported continuing with her ultradian self-hypnosis sessions. In her words, "I want to stay thin, and don't want to be my old size."

In another case, participant four was a 58 year-old, married, female office worker. She scored non-self-actualizer on the POI, moderate state anxiety, high trait anxiety, mild-moderate depression, and high stress symptoms (thoughts, emotions, physical symptoms). She scored high on hypnotizability. Her stated goal was how to deal with a very disempowering work situation. At pretreatment (before the self-hypnosis sessions), her nasal cycle recordings showed either a predominance of one nostril constantly open with no alternation to the opposite side or both nostrils were congested. According to yogic breathing practices, this lack of alternation between nostrils is a very unhealthy condition. Note her depression, anxiety, and stress symptom scores above.

A review of her comments over the course of the 12 weeks showed an increasing feeling of calm, happiness, and equanimity in dealing with the very difficult people in her work setting. She gained an understanding of their behaviors, and she felt more in control of her responses to them as a result. Overall, at debriefing, participant four said she felt "transformed." At first, she reported that she didn't think anything was happening. Then, she found certain events and insights catalyzed one another.

At week 12, her nasal cycle recordings showed a movement toward a more regular cycle, alternating between right and left and vice versa, as compared to the pre-treatment baseline measures. While her POI score remained stable, her trait anxiety decreased substantially, her depression score dropped from mild-moderate to normal, and her stress symptoms also decreased.

In summary, the ultradian cycles analyzed in this case study approach became more normalized with the practice of ultradian self-hypnosis (which supports Rossi's[22] hypothesis), and persons who are highly hypnotizable showed the most change. There were varying reductions in levels of anxiety, depression, and stress symptoms. While the level of self-actualization is a more enduring measure, anxiety, depression, and stress symptoms appear to be more modifiable with the practice of self-hypnosis. A naturalistic approach to hypnosis did serve to regulate the ultradian nasal cycles.

Since the participant or client is accessing the unconscious without external suggestions and without the presence of the therapist, it is advisable to use this method of self-hypnosis with high functioning, educated, insight-oriented clients. It is important that the client is disciplined and can incorporate this type of practice into his/her own lifestyle. I have found this approach successful in the treatment of some anxiety disorders and mild-to-moderate personality types of obsessive-compulsive behaviors.

Conclusions

There are many theories of hypnosis yet each contributes to our overall understanding of this remarkable phenomenon. In my clinical work, I have found success in using ultradian self-hypnosis with high-functioning, motivated adults. Rather than posing external suggestions other than comfort to the client, and letting his or her unconscious do the work, in this approach the client poses his or her own problem to the unconscious, and the unconscious proceeds on its own course. This ebb and flow of receptivity and attention, and the timing of the hypnotic induction to the more receptive phase of an ultradian cycle, makes intuitive sense. Erickson fostered a trust in one's own unconscious. He said, "If you go into an auto-hypnotic trance, you must trust your own unconscious to pick the right thing for you to do." Rossi[24] proposes that a person needs to allow his or her unconscious to do its own work, without verbal suggestions which may distort the total personality's needs.

Perhaps as this ultradian self-hypnotic approach sets the process of balanced breathing into motion, it actually accesses the sixth chakra of intuitive knowledge (with its balance of the right and the left, the ida and pingala). The mechanism remains a mystery. Whether ultradian self-hypnosis simply accesses other transpersonal parts of the person usually outside of his or her awareness still needs further investigation. What does seem to be operating is a deepening of the breath, a regulation of biological rhythms, and an improvement in anxiety, depression, and stress symptoms. Without definitively knowing the operative mechanisms of this technique, the results presented here are quite remarkable. Rigorous scientific investigations may yield more understanding of ultradian cycles, and their possible links to hypnotic phenomena. Hypnosis, the transpersonal, and Eastern perspectives continue to be fascinating areas of study. They point us to more hidden realms and to the frontiers of human possibility.

References

1. Ajaya, S., *Psychotherapy east and west: a unifying paradigm*, Honesdale, PA, Himalayan International Institute of Yoga Science and Philosophy, 1983.
2. Arpita, The role of breathing in current clinical interventions, *Res. Bull. Himalayan Int. Inst.*, 4(1), 22–31, 1982.
3. Ballentine, R., Nasal function and energy, in *Science of breath: A practical guide*, S. Rama, R. Ballentine, and A. Hymes, Eds. , 57–87, The Himalayan International Institute of Yoga Science and Philosophy, Honesdale, PA, 1979.
4. Bhatnagar, S., *Innertuning therapy*, SRI Centre International, New York, 1980.
5. Bucke, R.M., *Cosmic consciousness: a study in the evolution of the human mind*, E.P. Dutton, New York, 1923.
6. Carrington, P., *Bodily rhythms, cosmic rhythms, and human well-being*, SRI Centre International, New York, 1986a.
7. Erickson, M.H. and Rossi, E.L., *Experiencing hypnosis: therapeutic approaches to altered states*, Irvington, New York, 1981.
8. Ferguson, M., *The aquarian conspiracy: personal and social transformation in the 1980s*, J.P. Tarcher, Los Angeles, 1980.
9. Friedman, S., A psychophysiological model for the chemotherapy of psychosomatic illness, *J. Nervous and Mental Dis.*, 166(2), 110–116, 1978.

10. Halberg, F., Chronobiology, *Ann. Rev. Physiol.*, 31, 675–725, 1969.

11. Iyengar, B.K.S., *Light on pranayama: the yogic art of breathing*, Crossroad, New York, 1987.

12. James, W., The varieties of religious experience, in C.T. Tart, *States of consciousness*, Psychological Processes, El Cerrito, CA, 1975, 55–56.

13. Kleitman, N., Basic rest-activity cycle in relationship to sleep and wakefulness, in *Sleep: Physiology and pathology*, A. Kales, Ed., Lippincott, Philadelphia, 1969, 33–38.

14. Lad, V., *Ayurveda: The science of self-healing*, Lotus Press, Santa Fe, 1984.

15. Naitoh, P., Chronobiologic approach for optimizing human performance, in *Rhythmic aspects of behavior*, F.M. Brown and R.C. Graeber, Eds., Lawrence Erlbaum Associates, Hillsdale, NJ, 1982, 41–103.

16. Nuernberger, P., *Freedom from stress: a holistic approach*, Himalayan International Institute of Yoga Science and Philosophy, Honesdale, PA, 1981.

17. Osowiec, D.A., Ultradian rhythms in self-actualization, anxiety, and stress-related somatic symptoms, *Dissertation Abstracts International*, 53, 04B, University Microfilms 92-24529, 1992.

18. Osowiec, D.A., Self-hypnosis and ultradian rhythms: Some case studies, In D.A. Osowiec and E.L. Rossi, *Pathways of Mind-Body Healing*, paper presented at the 35th Annual Scientific Meeting of the American Society of Clinical Hypnosis, New Orleans, LA, March 1993.

19. Rama, S., The science of prana, in *Science of breath: a practical guide*, S. Rama, R. Ballentine, and A. Hymes, The Himalayan International Institute of Yoga Science and Philosophy, Honesdale, PA, 1979, 89–143.

20. Rama, S., Ballentine, R., and Ajaya, S., *Yoga and psychotherapy: the evolution of consciousness*, The Himalayan International Institute of Yoga Science and Philosophy, Honesdale, PA, 1976.

21. Rama, S., Ballentine, R., and Hymes, A., *Science of breath: a practical guide*, The Himalayan International Institute of Yoga Science and Philosophy, Honesdale, PA, 1979.

22. Rossi, E.L., Hypnosis and ultradian cycles: a new state(s) theory of hypnosis? *Am. J. Clinical Hypnosis*, 25(1), 21-32, 1982.

23. Rossi, E.L., Hypnosis and ultradian rhythms, in B. Zilbergeld, G. Edelstien, and D. Araoz, Eds., *Hypnosis: questions and answer*, Norton, New York, 1986b, 17–21.

24. Rossi, E.L., *The psychobiology of mind-body healing: new concepts of therapeutic hypnosis*, Rev. ed., Norton, New York, 1993.

25. Tart, C.T., *States of consciousness*, Psychological Processes, El Cerito, CA, 1975.

26. Werntz, D.A., Cerebral hemispheric activity and autonomic nervous function, *Dissertation Abstracts International*, 42, 06B, University Microfilms DDJ81-25444, 1981.

27. Werntz, D.A., Bickford, R.G., Bloom, F.E., and Shannahoff-Khalsa, D.S., Alternating cerebral hemispheric activity and the lateralization of autonomic nervous function, *Human Neurobiol.*, 4, 225–229, 1983.

28. Werntz, D.A., Bickford, R.G., and Shannahoff-Khalsa, D.S., Selective hemispheric stimulation by unilateral forced nostril breathing, *Human Neurobiol.*, 6, 165–171, 1987.

For further study:

Himalayan International Institute of Yoga Science and Philosophy
RR 1, Box 400
Honesdale, PA. 18431
(570) 253-5551
1-800-822-4547

The business office has a listing of certified yoga teachers across the country.

Yoga International Magazine (see Teacher's Directory)
R.R.1, Box 407
Honesdale, PA 18431
(570) 253-4929
Fax: (570) 253-6360

A reputable yoga center in your area.

chapter seven

Animal imagery and the Personal Totem Pole Process®

Eligio Stephen Gallegos

The theoretical underpinning of the Personal Totem Pole® process involves the assumption that each human being is primarily an awareness. This awareness, in order to function optimally, needs to have full input from all modes of knowing. There are four modes of knowing: thinking, sensing, feeling, and imagery. Each of these modes of knowing is unique in itself and is not reducible to any of the other three. The natural state of these modes of knowing is to function in harmony with one another.

Adam and Eve lived in perfect harmony in the Garden of Eden. The masculine and the feminine lived without conflict, compatible, and fully integrated. Their world was whole and undivided, a rich river of the flow of being in experience. This was a world of abundance. Humans and animals lived peaceably together. The lion lay down with the lamb. Judgment, conflict, and polarization were unknown.

In this place, one thing only was forbidden: eating of the apple of the knowledge of good and evil. But how can one act be denied in a world where all aspects of life are in harmony? When the serpent enticed Eve to eat the forbidden fruit, she did so willingly, because, as the feminine principle, she knew the world through feeling and imagery: curiosity, the instinct to integrate all aspects of experience, and a sense of adventure. Once she had eaten, the masculine principle was introduced into the Garden: knowing through thinking and the propensity to polarize.

We have replayed this myth in our own upbringing, time and time again, generation after generation. Once we leave the world of infancy, where all parts of ourselves and our world are integrated, and instead begin knowing through thinking, then we are thrust into the actions of polarizing and

0-8493-2237-5/00/$0.00+$.50
© 2000 by CRC Press LLC

judging, and of separating concepts (in fact, polarization is the basis of conceptualization). All that has previously existed in harmony and without conflict begins to be experienced and evaluated in terms of opposites; one pole is accepted, the other rejected. Then Heaven and Earth are split asunder, God and the Devil cannot co-exist, and we begin living by division, conflict, and separation.

The "medical model," scientifically based on objective reality, treats two of these modes of knowing as valid (thinking and sensing) and invalidates or devalues the other two (feeling and imagery).[12] It does this by presuming that feeling and imagery can be understood or known through the medium of thinking and sensing (for example, by reducing all knowing to "brain function": the brain, being physical, is at the seat of who we are and we will eventually have the theory that explains its relation to how we function). The Personal Totem Pole process on the other hand, recognizes the uniqueness of each of the four modes of knowing, none of which is ultimately reducible to any of the other three. So the theory of the Personal Totem Pole process, although stated verbally and put forth through the thinking mode, supports the uniqueness and the autonomy of each of the other three modes of knowing. This is a fundamental difference between the Personal Totem Pole process and the medical model.

We live in a culture that systematically teaches us that the scientific orientation is the ultimate explanation. Thus what we are taught carries within itself the view that although sensing and logical thinking are valid ways of knowing, feeling and imagery are not. The Personal Totem Pole process understands this division in itself to be a form of injury, a form of separating thinking and sensing from feeling and imagery in our understanding of who we are. Furthermore, this "understanding of who we are" constitutes an identity, and the identity itself is injured in that it has learned to reject (or at least seriously question) part of the organic nature of the individual. The rejection (or questioning) takes place primarily in the mode of knowing that we call thinking. The healing of this cultural injury can be brought about through learning to honor feeling and imagery as valid modes of knowing. Imagery, the oldest and deepest mode of knowing, carries within itself the qualities of integration as a dimension of its function. Thus the function of the Personal Totem Pole therapist or guide is to help the individual return to a full relationship with imagery as a mode of knowing.

Once the relationship is honored, then knowing through imagery introduces experiences which over time return the individual to a balanced and unified organic functioning. This return is frequently comprised of the experiences of discovering and healing the injuries which originally resulted in the separation of thinking/sensing from imagery/feeling, but it also involves the experiences of discovering and filling out inherent positive qualities and capabilities of the individual that have not yet found full expression in his or her life. So the Personal Totem Pole process not only undertakes the healing of old injuries but also of helping the individual move into wholeness and a fullness of being that may not have been previously evident.

The Personal Totem Pole Process begins with the premise that there are four fundamental ways, or "windows," of knowing: thinking, sensing, feeling, and imagery.[4,5] This is different from C. G. Jung's four functions of consciousness[7] which he named thinking, sensing, feeling, and intuition. The difference, however, is not as great as it may seem. In Jung's writings it is evident that his intuition arrived through his window of imagery. Intuition is a way of knowing something for which there is no logical precedent, but in the perspective of the Personal Totem Pole Process, intuition can occur through any of the four modes of knowing. The primary focus of the Personal Totem Pole Process is on knowing through imagery.

Thinking and sensing have long been considered the only valid ways of knowing in Western science and most of us in modern society unconsciously behave as if this were true. Medicine, most psychotherapy, education, and many other disciplines would have us believe that humans are composed of objective parts, interrelated like parts of a machine that just happens to be organic. Accompanying this view is the belief that we can be modified, either positively or negatively, by removing, changing, or influencing these discrete parts.

Feeling and imagery are ways of knowing that integrate the many diverse parts of us, rather than separating them. However, because we are unaccustomed to this point of view, we are often uncomfortable with ways of knowing that challenge the thinking and sensing windows we have been taught to rely on for our truth about the world. As a result, we often try to comprehend feeling and imagery not on their own terms, but from the point of view of thinking and sensing, a skewed perspective that often ignores or dishonors the unique realms of feeling and imagery. Because feeling and imagery do not fit the familiar paradigms of thinking and sensing, they are denigrated by being deemed as invalid ways of knowing. The Personal Totem Pole Process honors feeling and imagery as unique ways of knowing that have the capacity to instruct us in their dimensions if we are but willing to venture into a relationship with them without prejudice and without trying to force them into paradigms of thinking and sensing.[6]

The view of modern physicists, as well as the views of most mystics, is that matter is comprised of energies. The direct equivalence of matter and energy was formally posed by Albert Einstein in his famous equation, $E = mc^2$. The Personal Totem Pole Process acknowledges that human beings are comprised of energies of infinite variety and complexity and helps them enter into a relationship with themselves at this level. One way to know these diverse energies fully and deeply is to enter freely into the window through which imagery presents itself to us. Just as we have to open our eyelids in order to see with our physical senses, we must open the eye of imagery to see what it has to show us, something we do quite naturally when we dream or create even the simplest works of art.[1] The Personal Totem Pole Process encourages us to enter into a relationship with these diverse energies or dimensions of ourselves, rather than trying to control, dominate, or manipulate them.

The typical Personal Totem Pole Process session involves initial deep relaxation of the client. This is done in order to enable a focus on the dimension of imagery rather than being preoccupied with thinking and evaluating. If thinking and evaluating are particularly prominent, they are invited to stand to one side and to learn, while imagery takes the fore for a change. The Personal Totem Pole Process does not involve itself in specifically attempting to induce trance states. It considers that a trance state is a state of narrowed awareness and that this is already the state of the vast majority of civilized people, as we have all been thoroughly conditioned to allow the description or the intellectual map to dominate the world that we are willing to perceive.

In the first stage of the Personal Totem Pole Process, the energies that make up the core of the human energy system, known in the Orient as the chakras,[8] are specifically invited to show themselves in the form of animals.[2,3] Thus, seven animals, one for each chakra, come forth one at a time, and the client is invited to enter into a relationship with them. The client can speak with them, provide for their needs, go on journeys with them to memories, emotions, sources of conflict or illness, or aspects of creativity, or even to become them. In this way, clients gain access to aspects of themselves that are usually hidden or known only partially and incompletely through thinking or sensing. The animals of imagery are alive and independent; we do not own them or have control over them. Yet because they represent parts of ourselves, they are very willing to support us in who we truly are, not in who we have learned to become for social survival or acceptance.

When the animals appear to us, they embody the status of the chakra from which they arose. For example, someone who was hurt in a love relationship may see in the heart chakra a bird with a broken wing. As the client helps the bird heal its injury, the client's emotional injury is healed as well.

It is fascinating that the animals invariably typify the chakra energies as they are classically understood, even though the client may have no knowledge whatsoever of the chakra system. In other words, the chakra at the crown of the head is involved in spiritual matters, the chakra at the forehead is related to thinking, the throat is involved with communication, the heart with love and compassion, the solar plexus with action and power, the belly with passion and emotion, and the chakra at the base of the spine with groundedness and relation to the earth. I hesitate to provide examples of these because of the human capacity for self comparison and evaluation. One of the great difficulties we have had in coming to know who we are is that we have been given descriptions almost from the day of our birth about who it is we are supposed to be,[9,10,11] and we have tried to fit ourselves to others' ideas about us instead of approaching ourselves openly and discovering through our own experiences who is this being called "myself." However, the chakra animals allow us to do this in a beautiful and remarkable manner. Even so, it is not up to either the client or the therapist to attempt to predict these dimensions intellectually; our true option is to discover them and to learn from them.

As we return to the place where we may know ourselves openly, our individual Garden of Eden, profound healing usually occurs, for it is typically through injury or in response to threat that we have been separated from our true center and that we have diminished our wholeness. The instances of pain and injury that the animals evoke and that require healing are frequently ones that the person has completely forgotten about until the imagery reintroduced them. So the Personal Totem Pole Process helps us enter a way of knowing that is older and more organic than our intellectual knowing. By healing the injuries we have sustained, we can return to our natural healthy state.

The Personal Totem Pole Process helps this journey of self-fulfillment and healing to advance even further by inviting the animals from all seven chakras to come together to form a council. Sometimes the animals have been separate from one another for many years; occasionally some animals are unable or unwilling to get along with others. In council the animals initiate the process of healing their relationship with one another, coming back into balance, and guiding the growth, healing, and fulfillment of the individual.

It is important to emphasize that this growth is not determined by the theoretical structures of the therapist, but by the ongoing relationship that the individual develops and maintains with his or her own deep imagery process. Some therapeutic methods that utilize imagery are highly intrusive and I wish to definitively differentiate the Personal Totem Pole Process from these. The imagery that arises spontaneously from the deep parts of our imagery has its own intelligence and carries an orientation of healing and moving toward wholeness. This is a highly organic process and it happens at its own pace and in its own time frame.

Our natural relationship with it was originally one of trust and welcoming it as a valued dimension of our being. When the therapist attempts to impose an image that is prepared beforehand, what I call canned imagery, this can occasionally have a negative effect, or at the least be intrusive upon a process that is natural to each individual. The Western attitude of changing and fixing does not bring a person back into wholeness, but serves to maintain the perspective that intrusion into one's deepest process is the only available way. It was such intrusion in the first place that brought about most of the injuries that are encountered in psychotherapy. Psychotherapy needs to honor the natural healing and wholeness of the client rather than becoming a perpetrator of injurious intrusiveness. The ultimate goal of the Personal Totem Pole Process is to arrive at a harmonious interaction between all dimensions of an individual, so he gains a deep respect for his own process, the process underlying not only his thoughts and behavior, but his feelings and ultimate wholeness.

One of the most damaging lessons we learn, under the guise of socialization, is that some other authority's ideas of who we are supposed to be are more valid than our own. What is fundamentally a theft of our own individual ways of knowing happens regularly and consistently from the time we are infants, with parents, with teachers, and with therapists who begin with a theoretical assumption or who insist on interpreting the individual according to preconceived notions. Such methods perpetuate the injury under the guise of healing it. The only true healing we can offer is to assist another person to come to a place where he stands firmly gounded in his own ways of knowing, where he can tell his own story with his own experience as the source of that story.

The Personal Totem Pole Process is an orientation that helps heal the division between thinking and imagery by promoting a relationship between our personal identity and the animals that come to us in imagery. The animals help our identity grow so that it comes closer to encompassing the full humanness that is our birthright, rather than an identity whose function is social interaction and social survival. The animals bring us closer to participating directly with that energy that is the core substance of our being, and it is an energy no different from the energy that once filled the mythical Garden of Eden and still fills the universe. The animals quickly show us two things: one, that we have been stuck in the places of our deepest injuries, and in one way or another have been living these injuries over and over through a strange conjunction of attempting to avoid the circumstances that brought them about and, at the same time, unknowingly inflicting them on those we are closest to. And secondly, imagery shows us that the natural movement of being alive is to return to a place where the injuries are healed, a place, moreover, where the injury may be transformed into extraordinary strength.

The Personal Totem Pole Process views all separation as an injury. Therefore, the natural path of healing is toward greater and greater integration. Healing brings us back to the Garden of Eden. Injury drives us away from it. The great value of having been injured is that, with the healing, we have knowledge of that hurt place as well as the healed place that replaces it, so we can hold the space within which another person can heal, without condemning the injury or judging the person's need to protect himself from further injury.

The Personal Totem Pole Process has been employed successfully in working with children as well as adults. It is cross-cultural and works at all levels of educational achievement. It has been used in prisons and in hospitals, with physical ailments and addictions, with spiritual and emotional problems. It is a method that is completely natural to who we are. The Personal Totem Pole Process returns us to a deep dimension whose natural function is to maintain us in health and to help us grow into our fullness – in other words, to help us return to our own Garden of Eden.

Case study

One of my clients was a woman who I will call Jane. Before I became her therapist, she had been in group therapy for five years, since first experiencing a nervous breakdown for which she had been hospitalized. Her symptoms were depression, self-negation, and extreme suicidal tendencies. Her previous therapists had encouraged her to enter into non-suicide contracts with them and she admitted to me at the end of our therapy that she had restated the contract to herself almost daily in order to keep from attempting suicide.

Jane was 34 years old, divorced, with two children. Her manner was intense and she had a high pitched voice. The first time I met with her was in a group setting. She expressed a fear of me. I assured her that I respected her and trusted her ability to grow, and that I would do nothing to threaten or pressure her, which she accepted. She told me at the time that she hated herself because she wasn't perfect. I told her that I felt each human being was a beautiful flower deep inside. She replied that she was sure there was no flower within herself. I had the group do a visualization to get in touch with the inner flower. Jane expressed surprise at what she had seen: a tiny baby.

At our first individual session I heard more of her history. She had grown up on a remote ranch in northern Wyoming. Her mother was dominating, usually angry, and defensive. Jane felt she had never been good enough for her mother and that she had not been wanted from the time she was born. Her older sister had a personality similar to that of her mother. Her father was passive and quiet.

She said she felt like she was nothing; her existence was a deep dark well with a lid over it. The only delight she had experienced in her early life was when her father took her hunting or fishing with him. Although he seldom said anything, on these occasions she felt that he truly cared for her. When I asked if she could give each of these little girls a different name, this one she called "Richness." The other's name was "Nothing."

She also expressed a tendency to want to withdraw into a corner where she would be safe. I assured her she was free to retreat to the corner whenever she wished, as she was also free to come out of that corner. I encouraged her to practice both of these movements so they could both become voluntary.

At our next individual session I asked her to place the chairs in the room to represent the positions of family members at home. Her mother's and sister's chairs were placed in the center of the room; her own and her father's were placed in two corners. She told me that as a newborn baby her position had been at the center of the room. I invited her to sit in that position now. When she did, she immediately felt jealousy from her mother and sister. As she removed herself to the corner her father also moved to a corner in silent support of her.

In the following group session I used guided imagery to bring the members of the group into contact with their chakra animals. The animal in Jane's forehead (intellectual/intuitive) was a giant eagle. Jane was standing below it and could only see its legs and lower body. Its first words were to tell her how dumb and stupid she was. She was shocked by this and asked it why it was saying such things. It replied that it wanted to give her an example of what she does to herself.

The animal in her throat (communication) was a weasel. Jane felt demeaned at this, but there was an understanding that perhaps she used communication in attempts to weasel out of some things. The animal in her heart (love/compassion) was a dead dog encrusted with a fungal growth, lying on a stone slab in a cave. The dog had apparently been dead for a considerable length of time. Jane was visibly shaken at the encounter with the dead dog.The animal in her solar plexus (power) was a white bird in a cage. The bird asked Jane to open the door and release it. She did as requested and when it emerged from the cage it turned into a large dragon, roaring in anguish. Jane, terrified, immediately seized it, shoved it back into the cage and closed the door, whereupon it once again became a white bird. The animal in her belly (emotion/passion) was a small fuzzy bear. He reached inside of Jane and removed a small blue stone. As he held it up, a soft blue glow emanated from the stone which illuminated the entire room with a good feeling. Her grounding animal was a playful porpoise.

I asked Jane to invite her animals to gather together so that they themselves could assess the circumstances and decide on what action needed to be taken. She went to each animal and invited it, but when she came to the white bird it told her that it would have to be released from its cage in order to attend the council meeting. She reluctantly opened the cage door and allowed it to emerge. Again it turned into a dragon, roaring loudly. Jane suddenly became aware that it wasn't roaring so much as wailing, wailing because the dog was dead.

As the animals gathered, they met in the cave and formed a circle around the dead dog as it lay on the stone slab. As they stood there, Jane among them, she suddenly became aware of the presence of a small baby and a fifteen year old boy. I watched as she burst into uncontrolled sobbing.

"That's the baby that I was pregnant with when I was nineteen! I had an abortion! I shouldn't have done that! It was completely wrong! It was terrible of me to have the abortion! I shouldn't have done it! I shouldn't have done it!"

This was the first I had known of the abortion.

She knew that the fifteen year old boy was the baby had it been allowed to live. The boy turned to her and said, "It's okay. I'm content where I am. You did what you needed to do at the time and I'm not angry at you. Now you need to accept the fact that you had the abortion and not judge yourself."

She again burst into tears. "No! It was wrong! I shouldn't have done it! I shouldn't have done it! I killed that little baby!"

The boy and all the animals now looked at her compassionately but firmly and said, "You need to accept the fact that you had the abortion."

Again she railed, "I can't! I can't! It was wrong of me to do that!"

Calmly and firmly, they reiterated, "You need to accept it."

There was no coercion on the part of the animals, and no attempt to force Jane in any way. Yet they were firmly of one mind.

After a bout of prolonged crying Jane quietly said, "All right. I accept it. I had the abortion."

At this the dog suddenly returned to life. It's coat became sleek and shiny, and it stood up and moved to Jane's side. The dragon stopped its wailing. And the weasel turned into a swan.

Her voice was no longer high pitched, but had a new softness as she said, "I guess I've condemned myself enough. I was only a kid." All of the animals celebrated the dog's return to life, and the baby and boy were gone.

Jane was astonished and deeply moved.

With a surprisingly small amount of further work Jane's depression of the previous five years lifted. It was then that she confessed to me that during those five years she had made a pact with herself daily that she would not commit suicide on that day. It is obvious now that a major source of her depression was the hatred that she felt toward herself for having undergone the abortion. As I stated previously, I had known nothing about her abortion and I don't know that her previous therapist had known anything about it. The beautiful thing was that the chakra animals took her immediately to that event at her first meeting with them. Furthermore, they also undertook the healing that was necessary. They were able to bring her to the place where she was willing to stop the self hatred and just accept what she had done.

Two other energies were related to her depression. One was the caging of her solar plexus animal, the white bird/dragon. The solar plexus energy is sometimes referred to as the power center, but it is involved with action, with doing. Jane's "doing" was her self hatred, and when that ceased, the dragon stopped its wailing. The other energy was her throat chakra, the weasel. The throat energy is involved with expression, not just talking but all forms of expression including painting and music. Again, when the self hatred ceased, the weasel became a swan. Fast upon this transformation her voice changed. The immediacy of such a change is startling, and I have encountered this numerous times. What this says is that when an animal undergoes a change there is a corresponding change in the behavior of the client, and a change of some sort at the physical level.

Concluding remarks

Although this case study involves the healing of an emotional injury, this is only the initial aspect of the Personal Totem Pole Process. After healing has occurred, and in fact as it is proceeding, the more necessary aspect of being human is growing fully and gathering oneself into wholeness. Jung spoke of these processes as the processes of individuation and of transcendence. The Personal Totem Pole Process systematically carries the client through these processes at a pace appropriate to the nature of the individual, not a pace imposed by the theoretical assumptions or interpretations of the therapist.

In training therapists in this process as I have for the past ten years, it has become evident that the extent of the therapist's healing and growth determines the limit to which he can accompany and support the client. A common occurrence I have observed is that when the animals take a client into an old injury, if a similar injury has been sustained by the therapist and not yet healed, the therapist will tend to become overinvolved in the client's process, frequently to the point of intruding into the process rather than supporting the client in his relationship with the animals. Thus it is imperative for a therapist to grasp every opportunity to do his own healing and growing, for this is the preparation necessary for accompanying the client as far as the client can go.

References

1. Eliade, M., *Shamanism: archaic techniques of ecstasy*, Princeton, Bollingen, 1964.
2. Gallegos, E. S., *Animal imagery, the chakra system, and psychotherapy*, J. Transp. Psych., 1983, 15(2), 125–136.
3. Gallegos, E. S., *The Personal Totem Pole: animal imagery, the chakras, and psychotherapy*, 2nd ed., Moon Bear Press, Velarde, NM, 1990.
4. Gallegos, E. S., *Animals of the Four Windows: Voices: the art and science of psychotherapy*, 1990, 26(1), 49-61.
5. Gallegos, E. S., *Animals of the Four Windows: integrating the four modes of knowing: thinking, sensing, feeling, and imagery*, Moon Bear Press, Velarde, NM, 1992.
6. Hillman, J., *Re-Visioning Psychology*, Harper & Row, New York, 1975.
7. Jung, C. G., *Psychological Types*, Vol. 6, Collected Works of C. G. Jung, Princeton University Press, Princeton, NJ, 1957.
8. Motoyama, H., *Theories of the Chakras*, Theosophical Publishing House, Wheaton, IL, 1981.
9. Miller, A., *The Drama of the Gifted Child*, Basic Books, New York, 1981.
10. Miller, A., *For Your Own Good*, Farrar, Strauss & Giroux, New York, 1983.
11. Miller, A., *Thou Shalt Not Be Aware*, Farrar, Strauss & Giroux, New York, 1984.
12. Watkins, M., *Waking Dreams*, 3rd ed., Spring, Dallas, 1984.

For further study:

The Personal Totem Pole Process
Box 468
Velarde, NM 87582

chapter eight

Ericksonian hypnosis and meditation*

Steven Wolinsky

Trances are often a necessary means of surviving and negotiating the physical universe. They are like tunnels walked through in order to maneuver and focus in the world. Some trances are functional and pleasing; others are dysfunctional and pathological. Some trances will be in alignment with one's goals, while others will be impediments. What I call Deep Trance Phenomena are, at one and the same time, a means of survival for the overwhelmed child and the core of symptom structure for the coping adult. Those trance phenomena that create adult symptomatology usually have their origins in childhood patterns of experience.

Most of us automatically (or "unconsciously") recreate states of consciousness from the past as trance phenomena in the present. Many states of awareness involve some combination of Deep Trance Phenomena; any state that is problematic can be assumed to contain one or more trance phenomena. The task of the psychotherapist therefore becomes one of dehypnotizing the client: awakening the client's awareness to the deep trance that is being recreated from the original family context and which continues to function, unnoticed, as the invisible "glue" of the client's current daily symptom complex.

In essence, this awakening amounts to counting one's self in the therapy. Most forms of psychotherapy do not really count the person as a creative self; he or she is viewed as a product of all the other factors that are counted, feelings, thoughts, associations, problems, body sensations, muscle tonus, memories, and dreams. But these are all only creations of the self behind the trance, not the person, and while this can seem like

---

* This chapter was excerpted from Stephen Wolinsky's book *Trances People Live: healing approaches in quantum psychology,* published by The Bramble Company, Norfolk CT, 1991.

unnecessary philosophizing, the shift in attitude toward seeing the client as a creative being is a major one.

There is a well-known story from the Hindu text, the Upanishads, that beautifully makes this point about forgetting to count the Self:

> There are ten men walking through the woods. They come upon a river, which they must cross. Because the current is so strong, they are afraid that some of them might be washed away, so they decide to hold hands and lock arms as they cross. This way, no one will get lost. They reach the other side and, just to be sure, they decide to count to verify that everyone has made it across.
>
> The first man counts 1,2,3,4,5,6,7,8,9. "Somebody is missing!" he shouts in alarm. The next person in line begins to count: 1,2,3,4,5,6,7,8,9! "Oh, no! Somebody is missing! Who did we lose?" Each person, in turn, counts the lot of them and comes up with only 9 people.
>
> Finally a sage comes by and, hearing the nature of their complaint, realizes their mistake. He counts them, one by one, and reaches 10. "You are the tenth one," the sage says to each.

How does this story translate in the therapy session? It means that the therapist learns to communicate with the creative being, the self, behind the trance. It is the self that can change the trance and hence the symptom. The reason therapy succeeds or fails is not always due to the skill of the therapist, or to the severity or tenacity of early traumas, nor is it always due to the trance states themselves. It can be due to the being as a creative self, "the tenth one."

A symptom can be thought of as the nonutilization of unconscious resources. When we are in a symptom state, we are not making use of inner resources that are normally available to us. This happens because the central characteristic of any trance state used to create the symptom is that it shrinks our focus of attention. Interestingly, Erickson viewed this as desirable: trance helped the person to narrow his focus of attention and become unaware of all extraneous stimuli and concerns. He then made use of this attentional constriction to heighten and consolidate the person's concentration on the problem at hand and to evoke unconscious resources.

Here, this can be seen as a paradox: the person has created a problem, which requires a shrinking of the focus of attention. At the same time, Erickson has the client shrink his or her focus of attention even more, in order to create a therapeutic trance state. I am suggesting that the reverse is also true: it is this very narrowing or shrinking of attention, as it functions in the symptomatic trance state, that locks the person into an automatic response pattern resulting in a non-utilization of unconscious resources.

For example, in the symptomatic trance state of an anxiety attack (pseudo-orientation in time), I shrink my focus of attention to such an extent that I feel totally cut off from the world. I move from an *inter*personal trance to an *intra*personal trance. I have no idea how to make the attack stop, and that sense of helplessness (age regression) escalates the anxiety and even further shrinks my ability to focus on anything but anxiety. I "don't see" the phone (negative hallucination) and I "forget" (amnesia) that I can pick it up and call a friend. I "forget" that I have had many periods of time that were completely free of anxiety attacks; I "forget " that I have had control over countless past situations in my life. All of these resources remain untapped by me as long as my intense self-to-self trance, with its shrunken focus of attention and the Deep Trance Phenomena of pseudo-orientation in time, age regression, negative hallucination and amnesia, remain intact. In this state, I imagine a very vivid and frightening future that is devoid of options and solutions and filled with the uncontrollable, assaultive sensations of anxiety attacks.

By asking clients to describe their symptoms while breathing and look-ing at me, I interrupt this sort of self-to-self trance of the symptom by placing them (via eye contact) in a self-to-other trance with me. This changes the context in which the symptom occurs and adds the therapist as a resource in present. (This is a common technique in Gestalt therapy and was demon-strated to me in 1975 by Eric Marcus, M.D. and Jack Rosenberg, Ph.D.) Erickson pointed out that the adult in present time has resources that the traumatized child did not have. By keeping the client focused in the present, she is able to take the present with her into the past. This differs from therapies which have the adult re-experience past traumas without the buffer of present-time resources. Therapists need to understand that the client survived the trauma and later created resources to cope with it. To pretend those resources are not currently present and that the client needs to relive the trauma without them, is to needlessly dramatize a situation again that no longer reflects the present.

What I call the "no-trance state," Ericksonian hypnotherapists call "ther-apeutic trance," and the Eastern meditative traditions call "meditation." We are all looking at a similar phenomenon, our most natural and optimal state-of-being, but through different lenses. In Asia water is called "paune," in Europe it is called "aqua," in the Middle East it is called "mai." It's the same substance, whatever you call it. In an analogous manner, the natural state, the no-trance state, the therapeutic trance state, and the meditative state are all different words describing a similar phenomenological experience. This natural state has no boundaries that separate the individual from the rest of the cosmos. It is transpersonal. Pain and problems arise only when we leave this state and identify ourselves with limiting ideas, with our symptoms, with our personality.

Meditation is often discussed in terms of three stages:

- dharana, which is the practice of concentrating on a fixed point
- dhyana, which is the point at which the focus of attention becomes an unbroken flow of concentration
- samadhi, which is a total cessation of the subject-object relationship

Samadhi occurs when the boundaries between the person who is concentrating and the object being concentrated upon disappear. As samadhi continues, dispassion follows; the individual loses all tendencies to become identified with the contents of the mind. Identity becomes transpersonal.

This is similar to being in a therapeutic trance wherein there is a free flow of associations without identification, attachment, or interruption. Thoughts, feelings, and emotions pass through the person without the ordinary damper of judgments or labels. In meditation, this experience occurs as the meditator witnesses the flow of mental contents without attaching to them.

To superimpose these terms on a Western framework, Erickson's hypnotherapeutric techniques constitute dharana, the means by which a person's attention was focused and narrowed, allowing the person to then slip into therapeutic trance, or dhyana meditation. What differentiates therapeutic trance from meditation is that in therapeutic trance, the mind and its contents are worked with — they are reframed, reassociated, utilized, reinterpreted, dissociated, and so on. In meditation the mind is simply observed without intervention. In therapeutic trance, a problem is being presented for change. In meditation, the only problem is one's identification with one's thoughts and experiences.

In what I am calling the no-trance state (also in samadhi and satori) there is a clear sense of non-identification (yogis call this dispassion); there is a sense of flow, a sense of perceptions coming and going, a sense of being and perceiving without judgment or identification. Erickson called his own taste of this experience "being in the middle of nowhere." By contrast, in trance states of identification we constrict our focus of attention and fuse with each and every occurrence in the day; our sense of self and well-being fluctuate commensurately.

The trance states we normally call feelings ("I feel good," "I feel bad," "I am being rejected") are the states in which attention is shrunken and focused, identified and attached. These are the states that breed symptomatology. This is what patients bring to you. The Ericksonian concept of the therapeutic trance is phenomenologically similar to the Eastern concept of meditation and samadhi. In that framework, this state of being is not a trance state at all; rather, it is the transcendence of limiting states of mind and being.

In the non-pathological trance state of meditation (pre-samadhi), and in the pathological trance state that produces symptomatology, and in the non-pathological excursions into various "common everyday trances," there is a narrowing of attention. The difference is, in the non-pathological trance states, the narrowing is voluntary and leads to an expanded awareness. I sit down to meditate by choice; I pick up needlepoint consciously and intentionally. In the symptomatic trance state, the narrowing is involuntary and the trance "pops up" and remains as the dominating characteristic. I stay in that state of shrunken attention and I identify with the contents of whatever I'm narrowing my focus of attention down to.

Perhaps this is an appropriate time to establish a context for this approach in relation to the field of psychotherapy in general and the Ericksonian model of hypnotherapy in particular. Erickson introduced the naturalistic/utilization approaches to trance work and therapy that have become the foundation for a paradigmatic shift in the entire field of psychotherapy. In my work with Ericksonian principles, I became convinced that his naturalistic approaches could be integrated with Eastern orientations and perspectives. The key puzzle pieces, trance states, interrupting patterns of response, and symptoms, were present in each. The differences between the two approaches arose in how each of these puzzle pieces related to the other.

In the Eastern view, trance states are continually coming and going; the purpose of meditating is to learn to develop some part of the awareness so that it can watch or observe the flow of the trances and the flow of consciousness. This observing part is thereby no longer identified with the ebb and flow of mental life. This process of observing or witnessing is used to create a therapeutic interpersonal context for change.

When I moved out of a focus on Eastern orientations and back into Western therapeutic approaches, I found myself drawn to the Deep Trance Phenomena of hypnosis. I had no conscious understanding of why I was so attracted to this particular facet of hypnotic work. I felt compelled to understand what Deep Trance Phenomena were on an experiential level and apart from their circumscribed use in hypnotherapy. What I realized was that trance states are a crucial part of the fabric of our daily life experience as well as of our symptomatology.

In the Ericksonian model, I learned that trance states could be induced or facilitated as a therapeutic intervention to interrrupt the symptom structure and access unconscious potentials and resources. In my breakthrough moment, those puzzle pieces came together in an entirely new pattern; I saw that although trance states can be used to evoke resources and change on an unconscious level, they can also be used and are used to *create* the symptomatology with which we all struggle. I saw that the person who brings his or her problems and symptoms to me is already in a trance state, and that it is this very trance state that is interrupting his or her experience of the present moment, blocking unconscious potentials and resources, and creating problems and symptoms. The therapeutic intervention then involves working with the trance state the person has already created (which dehypnotizes him or her), rather than inducing or facilitating another kind of trance that may or may not be pivotal to the patient's symptom structure.

There is a subtle but important difference between utilizing presenting behavior and the presenting trance: Erickson observed and utilized minimal cues of the presenting behavior in order to narrow and fixate attention and induce a trance. I am interested in observing and utilizing the presenting Deep Trance Phenomena that are creating the symptom. The immediate behavior may be secondary and derivative in relation to the underlying trance mechanisms that are ongoing. I utilize only what is presented as the symptomatic trances by having the client re-create it in present time.

The beginning stage of therapy for any problem or symptom is to help the person to break from identifying with the presenting issue. We need to have the new and different experience of discovering that we are more than or larger than the source of distress with which we are so typically identified. If I learn to move outside this misidentification so that I can view it, observe it, describe it, perhaps even write about it or paint it, in short, if I am the knower of the problem, then I am bigger than it. Simply put, it is not me. I am creating a larger context of selfhood, a transpersonal self, that allows me to observe and disidentify at the same time. The problem no longer takes up all my inner space; it is surrounded by a context of perception and awareness that begins to diminish the valence of the problem.

You are not that which passes through your consciousness; you are not your thoughts, your emotions, your ideas, memories, fears. Deep Trance Phenomena are the means by which you shrink your self down to these limited states, by which you erroneously identify with the belief that "I'm a loser," or "I'm not smart enough," or "I can't get close." Once you shrink your sense of self down to become this belief or that belief by identifying with it, you find yourself completely isolated inside the experience. There is no context to provide perspective or resources. Anything that you identifiy with is going to limit you by blocking out any other experience.

If there were only one key point to this chapter, it would be that you are not your problem; you are not your trance states which create your problem. You are the creator and the knower or perceiver of your problem. You are the being who chose particular responses to handle particular types of experiences; and you are the being who put those responses on automatic. That is the larger context that therapy must awaken in any person seeking a solution to a problem or a resolution of a symptom.

The mind is a library, and what you choose to experience in the course of a day is a product of you, the being behind the transient states of consciousness, standing in the library and retrieving particular sections. If you so choose, you can take the flashlight of your awareness into the history section, or the relationship section, or the business section, or the body section, and retrieve whatever you need. The point is, all the material is always there, but it can only be viewed if you choose to focus your mental flashlight on it.

In order for a therapist to be able to help a client discover himself as the transpersonal knower, the therapist (needless to say) needs to be beyond his own Deep Trance Phenomena. In other words, he needs to be well versed in the practice of self-observation, well able to "catch" his own misidentifications, and familiar with the sensation of shifting among identities rather than identifying with them. Perhaps an example from my own life will demonstrate this point.

About a year and a half ago I was in a very intense relationship with a woman. I thought things were going along wonderfully when, one night, I received a phone call from her. She said that "it was over!"

With those three words I felt myself deluged with anger and hurt. For half an hour I ranted and raved, feeling desolate and abandoned. Then a shift occurred and I "remembered" all I know about how such unpleasant states are created. I got a very clear picture of having gone to my mental library and turning my flashlight of awareness onto the section called "Rejection," whereupon I retrieved all the standard responses I had learned for that experience and fully identified with them. By identifying with them, I was recreating them in present time. Worse, the problem was automatically enlarged and amplified: by going into the library of my mind and retrieving all past experiences labelled "Rejection," I was experiencing a lifetime of accumulated events rather than simply the one in the present moment. Past was melded to present, with the future thrown in for dramatic effect (the "this is the story of my life" theme).

I then felt a tangible sensation of expansion occur as the misidentifications fell away. I let the body responses run their own course, realizing that particular sensations don't have to mean rejection, humiliation or hurt. I am the one who gives sensations one label or another. So I observed as my body experienced flushing, rapid breathing, and heart palpitations. I noticed how the waves of emotion I had been calling rejection also frequently accompanied sexual arousal, or excitement at a Celtics game, or any number of other pleasant experiences. I realized that we not only choose our responses, but perhaps more importantly, we choose the labels we give them. A rose by any other name is not a rose.

The moment you step outside of your problem to observe it, you create a larger context for it. Observing or witnessing thus becomes a key activity of therapy. I first came across the concept of witnessing in Eastern literature, in the Bhagavad Gita, where Krishna is described as the Eternal Witness. Krishna gives counsel to poor Arjuna, who represents all of us normal humans in life crises. Krishna teaches Arjuna how to interact with his states of consicousness so that they do not rule him by developing an awareness of his true nature as witness. The entire Gita revolves around the concept of the Eternal Witness as the means of disentangling ourselves from worldly perils.

From my Eastern perspective, it seemed to me that therapeutic trance was really a Western method of trying to establish a transpersonal witnessing consciousness. In hypnosis literature, the term dissociation is used to describe trance processes whereby one part of the individual steps back and looks at the overall situation. When dissociation is used therapeutically in hypnotic work, it is most often described as a means of splitting off or "depotentiating" the conscious mind from the unconscious.[2] The conscious mind is viewed as the interloper; the unconscious mind as the bearer of all the fruits.

On one hand, I view dissociation as an automatic defense whereby for example, you experience yourself floating at the top of the room in order to defend yourself against a molestation. On the other hand, dissociation means not associating with. When you can choose to fuse or associate with and choose to not associate with (dis-association), you have developed the ability to choose or not to choose to witness the content of your experience.

Witnessing, furthermore, is characterized by a subtle but important shift in focus. It does not involve a sense of splitting or depotentiating different regions of the mind. It is a unified experience of perception that allows and embraces without limiting and shrinking one's focus of attention. Emphasis is placed on the awareness of the self or being behind the ongoing activity, rather than on portioning out and labeling different aspects of mental functioning.

I'll finish with several clinical examples of how this witness consciousness, or disidentification with the personality, opens the door to healing. The first case illustrates that every experience can be a resource, even if it seems unlikely or impossible.

I treated a client who as a child had never been allowed to "just be blah." Her parents were, as she described them, "very zippity-do-dah," always up, always energized, and emoting about something. As an adult, she had a problem with chronic, mild depression, she seemed forever stuck in (age regressed to) the dreaded blah feeling. She needed to fully experience the forbidden state free of judgment, solely from the position of the witness. For her as an adult, the experience of feeling blah without judgment was wonderful. Instead of turning into a lingering depression, she had complete permission to just be. It is a grand paradox: as long as you evaluate blah-ness as being something bad that you shouldn't experience, you're constatnly going to resist it, which, in turn, keeps the blah-ness ever present.

The next case is a more detailed outline of how Deep Trance Phenomena can be recontextualized by using the interpersonal trance to elicit the witness state, and its attendant transpersonal healing resources.

A woman came to see me because she was experiencing acute anxiety from the fact that her divorce would be final in two weeks and she would "lose everything." Her statement of the problem was enough to tell me that her primary trance symptom was pseudo-orientation in time: projecting a catastrophic outcome in the future and experiencing it in present time. I began to work with this trance by asking her to continue to re-create it for me in as much detail as possible, beginning with her body posture.

Slowly, as she recited the negative suggestions she saw as descriptive of her future, her shoulders slumped forward, her knees drew in rigidly, she clasped her hands tightly together, and fixed her eyes on the ground. I asked her to breath and look at me as she continued, so she lifted her eyes, leaving her chin and head hanging in a downward position. In a faint, weak voice she began muttering, "He's going to get the house. He's going to get the savings account. He's going to get the certificate accounts. He's going to get the furniture."

I took over her internal dialogue by repeating her statements and asking her to repeat them also. Intensifying the dynamic that creates the symptom paradoxically helps the person move out of it into an expanded state. This patient proceeded to demonstrate this Ericksonian principle of "the symptom is the cure" perfectly. After several minutes of repeating her negative self-suggestions, she grew quiet and her body posture melted and softened. I asked her what she was experiencing, and after a deep sigh she responded, "I can see the light at the end of the tunnel." From my perspective, "taking over" the client's self-induced trance (by repeating the statements out loud) takes over the conscious mind and allows the resources ("the light at the end of the tunnel") to emerge.

I pursued her metaphorical description, associating it verbally with the pending divorce settlement and adding progressive suggestions that created a two week time frame. The two weeks were not experienced day by day, but as an undifferentiated mass of time that was emotionally and psychologically overwhelming. In such situations, I create a time-period as well as define clear, signposted steps to mark progress. Erickson has often commented that we tend to overlook our successes; much of what he did was to resurrect these successes and present them back to the patient so that he or she could appreciate and enjoy each step along the way.

In this case, I understood the client's statement about light at the end of the tunnel to verify her unconscious perception of a favorable outcome, and then took her back and forth, across a time period of 14 days and across a latticework of 14 steps. Each day was a step toward the light at the end of the tunnel (something like the "12 days of Christmas" theme) and held a particular accomplishment for her. I kept the suggestions very general so that her own unconscious resources could fill in the specifics. I also had her looking back at the 14 days, the 14 steps, from the perspective of having already arrived at the light at the end of the tunnel. I used suggestions that remained general to review each step's unique point and marveling at how all the steps coalesced into such a radiant unified light.

I let the suggestions set in silence for a few minutes and then asked her what she was feeling. She said, "I feel like a butterfly." I took her butterfly metaphor as another resource and utilized it in suggestions such as: "How nice it is to know you can be at step 14 and look back at step 11, and step 7, and even steps 3 and 1." For quite a while she experienced herself in trance flying back and forth, exploring each one of the steps.

My most salient objective with this client was to help her use her own trance choice of pseudo-orientation in time to create a pleasant future. I also wanted her to return to the present, keeping all the wonderful feelings of freedom she had experienced as a butterfly. I used the metaphor of the butterfly, which she had given me, to facilitate her ease in moving back and forth in time from the perspective of the free butterfly rather than the anxiety-ridden woman.

Editor's note: In this vignette, Dr. Wolinsky evoked an archetypal transpersonal image, the bright light, to facilitate this woman's healing. Chapter 3 of this book outlined a possible mechanism for this type of healing, involving life energy; this energetic process may help explain how this woman responded positively to treatment. But the key therapeutic step in this vignette is the patient's disidentification with her ego/personality, a step that came when she assumed the transpersonal witness position. This transition, or re-identification, allowed the healing mechanisms of the higher self (or the unconscious mind, as the Ericksonians call it) to enter into play.

References

1. Erickson, M. and Rossi, E., *Hypnotherapy: an exploratory casebook*, Irvington Press, New York, 1979.
2. Erickson, M. and Rossi, E., *Experiencing Hypnosis: therapeutic approaches to altered states*, Irvington Press, New York, 1981.
3. Fagan, J. and Shepherd, I., Eds., *Gestalt Therapy Now*, Harper and Row, New York, 1970.
4. Rossi, E. and Ryan, M., Eds., *Creative Choice in Hypnosis*, Vol IV, Irvington Press, New York, 1991.
5. Singh, J., *Vijnana Bhairava, or Divine Consciousness*, Motilal Bangrsida, Delhi, India, 1979.
6. Wolinsky, S., *Quantum Consciousness: the discovery and birth of quantum psycholology*, Bramble Company, Falls Village, CT, 1992.

For further training:

Quantum Psychology Institute
5600 Gibson SE, Suite 301
Albuquerque, NM 87108
(505) 254-1022

chapter nine

Jungian past life regression

Roger J. Woolger

Introduction: reincarnation in western thought

The notion that physical and psychological illnesses may be derived from the psychic residues of events in previous lives is accepted in a great many non-western cultures. The opening lines of the classic Buddhist text, the Dhammapada, sums up this view succinctly, "All that we are is the result of what we have thought." It hardly need be added that in the Buddhist world view, earlier thoughts can most certainly belong to earlier incarnations. In the West, however, Christianity had expunged all traces of reincarnational teachings from its dogma by the sixth century and orthodox Judaism has never laid any strong emphasis on it even though the Kabbalah, its esoteric or secret path, has an elaborate reincarnational doctrine taught to initiates into that tradition.

It is not until the nineteenth century that fully articulated doctrines of karma and reincarnation reappear among certain spiritualist groups in France, America, and England[14] notably the Theosophical writings of H.P. Blavatsky and Alice P. Bailey.[8] These have been a strong influence on the contemporary New Age movement where they have been reinforced more recently by the readings of the trance medium, Edgar Cayce.[16] From the perspective of contemporary biological and psychiatric science, however, the common view has largely remained that, strictly speaking, only constitutional predisposition towards depression and other organically based syndromes can be inherited; as for precise memories or mental contents, the opinion prevails, derived from the English empiricist philosopher John Locke, that the mind of an infant at birth is a "tabula rasa" or blank slate.[7]

In the psychoanalytic tradition one might expect that early explorations of the unconscious mind would have encountered past life memories, but among the great pioneers, Freud shied away from what he called "the flood tide of the occult"[13] clearly wishing to distance himself from scandals and charlatanism often associated with the practice of mediumship and the paranormal experimentation in that period. Nevertheless, there is in the annals of psychoanalysis one early follower of Freud who reported past life memories from his explorations of the unconscious mind using hypnosis, and that is a certain Colonel de Rochas who published a long forgotten study.[21] Possibly influenced by the French spiritualism of Alain Kardec, (1867) de Rochas found he was able to hypnotically regress patients back "before" their birth and to obtain, going still further backwards in time, memories of past lives, which seemed to arise in reverse historical sequence as alternately male or female.

The great Swiss psychiatrist, C.G. Jung, who broke with Freud, was much more given to the investigation of psychical phenomena; in fact, his doctoral thesis, "On the Psychology and Pathology of So-Called Occult Phenomena"[10] was a study of the channelings of a young medium. Jung however, assiduously avoided committing himself to any metaphysical interpretation of the phenomena encountered. Instead he regarded the spirit guides or controls that purportedly belonged to the previous lives of the medium to be secondary or subordinate personality fragments, that had been split off from the medium's ego personality and projected into a realm called spirit. Later, because of the many common features of these split off fragmentary personalities, Jung coined the term *archetype* to denote their universal features and dubbed the realm in which they dwelt the collective unconscious in order to avoid the question-begging term *spirit realm*. In Jung's little known 1938 lectures on the Yoga Sutras of Patanjali, he compares the Sanskrit concept *samskara*, which means roughly a psychic imprint or residue from a previous life, with his own concept of the archetype.[2] This line of thought was never developed and perhaps because of his persistent hostility to Theosophy he only came to a tentative acceptance of reincarnation as a psychic datum at the very end of his life.[27]

No further accounts of the use of hypnotherapy or psychoanalysis to explore 'past lives' are recorded in psychological literature of any kind for nearly half a century. It was not until the late 1950's that the subject of past lives being accessible to hypnosis and other techniques re-emerged. L. Ron Hubbard's enormously successful practice of Dianetics involved traveling backwards in time to other lives to find the engram, or original traumatic situation, behind any persistent current disturbance.[9] Hubbard's notion is actually very close to the yogic idea of the samskra. Unfortunately, despite its highly efficient methods, once Dianetics became absorbed into the Church of Scientology, it received very bad press for its rigidity and authoritarianism. For example, Winafred Lucas, a psychotherapist practicing in that era, deplored "the absence in the Dianetics work of awareness of the need for a therapeutic relationship."[18]

Also in the 1950s, two very different practitioners of hypnosis stumbled upon past life awareness. One was Morey Bernstein, who published the famous case of "Bridey Murphy," an 18th century past life personality who surfaced during hypnotic regression experiments with a friend.[1] Bernstein, a lawyer and an amateur hypnotist, had no training in therapy and was merely interested in the incredible historical detail of the memories. The case was and remains controversial, raising the common skeptical reaction that the so-called memories had been unconsciously overheard stories from the subject's childhood, a phenomenon known as cryptomnesia.[22]

The emergence of past life regression as a therapeutic modality

In England in 1967, the psychiatrist Denys Kelsey discovered he could regress patients both to prenatal memories and seeming past lives. He teamed up with the psychic and healer Joan Grant, who had already written a number of past life novels through what she termed *far memory,* a trance-like recall of her own previous lives. Because of Kelsey's medical credentials, his work was treated more seriously than Bernstein's was in America. Kelsey and Grant's book, *Many Lifetimes,*[15] remains a classic in the field.

With its opening to Eastern philosophy, meditation, and altered states of consciousness, some induced by LSD, the 1960s produced a change of climate, making past lives and reincarnation more generally acceptable. In fact, historians of the so-called New Age movement see reincarnation as a cornerstone of New Age philosophy and metaphysics.[17] It was then that Edgar Cayce's past life readings from the 1800s finally became widely known; channeled entities such as Jane Robert's "Seth" proclaimed past lives and multidimensional reality; Stanislav Grof's subjects who were regressed under LSD reported past life visions, and finally Jung, after considerable hesitation, chose to report encounters with past life material shortly before his death.[13]

A small but dedicated number of therapists struck by the economy and effectiveness of past life therapy began using regression in their practices. In California, Morris Netherton published his findings in *Past Lives Therapy*[20] as did Edith Fiore in *You Have Been Here Before.*[5] Interestingly Fiore was a hypnotherapist, while Netherton proclaimed that hypnosis was not only unnecessary to access past life memories, but that it might be contraindicated, since it dissociates the subject too much from the material. Instead Netherton employed affect laden phrases to help a client free associate back to a past life. In this, his method resembles Gestalt therapy practice, though Netherton disclaims any derivation from the work of Perls.

Independently in Germany, Thorwald Dethlefsen was using formal hypnosis to regress clients to past lives in psychotherapy, with startling results.[3] In a subsequent book, *The Challenge of Fate,*[4] Dethlefsen decided to drop formal hypnotic inductions, instead using altered state imagery to take clients into past life memories. At the same time in the Netherlands, Hans Ten Dam developed his own style of regression therapy[24] which led to the widespread acceptance of the technique in Holland. Later, a major training program in past life therapy was founded by four students of Ten Dam's, which is currently the largest in the world.

In the United States, an attempt has been made to synthesize Jungian, Reichian, and Gestalt practices with guided imagery and eastern concepts of the subtle bodies by the current author, Roger Woolger, in *Other Lives, Other Selves*.[28] This approach sees sub-personalities as past life manifestations to be psycho- dramatically and energetically cleared and integrated into the present personality. The psychiatrist Brian Weiss has made the hypnotherapy approach to regression widely known in his *Many Lives Many Masters*, while the prominent hypnotherapists Ernest Rossi and David Cheek have also written of encountering past lives during regression work.[23] In 1993 Winafred Lucas produced a two volume compendium *Regression Therapy*,[18] which is a state of the art summary of contemporary work in past lives, birth regression, as well as related and equally controversial topics such as sprit releasement (see Chapter 11 in this book for more details).

Finally, mention should be made of two prominent professional organizations that represent and promote past life therapy. One is the California-based Association for Past-Life Research and Therapy founded in 1980, which publishes *The Journal of Regression Therapy*, the other is the Dutch Foundation for Reincarnation Therapy, based in Amsterdam, which has an extensive training program for past life therapists and publishes a journal, *Cyclus*.

Imagining the body: the key to past life therapy

C.G. Jung developed a highly practical technique for working with his own dreams and visions.[11,13] He taught it to his own patients and trainees, and it is commonly used in Jungian analysis today. It consists primarily in sitting, as in meditation, and simply observing a fragment of a dream or hypnogogic image without any attempt to guide, control, or interfere with it. The aim is to allow the image to come to life of its own autonomous psychic energy, the ego letting go of all expectations, pre-suppositions, or interpretations. After a certain period of practice and initial coaching by the therapist, this inner image will start to move in some way, and the observing ego learns to participate in the story very much as the dream ego participates in normal dreaming. This waking dream ego is encouraged to encounter the imaginal situation as directly as possible, to avoid retreat and to fully allow any emotions such as fear, anger, sadness, eros, etc., to arise during the inner psychodrama. The ultimate goal of such practice, as both Jung and Roberto Assagiolo, (another early psychoanalyst who also formed his own school called, significantly, Psychosynthesis), is to work to integrate secondary or split off personality fragments into consciousness.

Jung's technique, which resembles other 'waking dream' practices,[26] has the invaluable effect of stimulating, focusing, and training the "inner senses" so that dreaming and waking meditation upon images becomes enormously enriched. This practice allows the unconscious psyche to express itself fully in its own language, imagery, and above all, to "dream the dream on" as

Jung put it on several occasions.[11] If and when "past life" images do arise (and there is no Jungian writing on this except van Waveren, see Reference 27), the practice would simply be to follow and participate in the imaginal story and in some instances to dialogue with inner figures that emerge. The key instruction remains to "stay with the image."

Powerful as this technique is, it proves inadequate for past life regression for a number of reasons. It does not distinguish between embodied and disembodied images, or between memories and dream stories, nor does it allow for the compensatory role of disembodied fantasy in imaginal situations where the ego is in apparent peril. This can be illustrated by the following excerpt from an active imagination session:

> I am walking through some dark woods. I see and hear
> some soldiers emerging from the trees. They are clearly
> planning to attack and rob me. They come closer. In
> terror I climb a tree. The tree turns into a stairway. I
> find myself in a childhood attic where I used to play
> with toy soldiers.

Taken as a psychotherapeutic exercise, this story can easily be seen as fantasy. The tree transforming into a stairway is clearly a fantasy event, and since the subject has no memories of being attacked by soldiers in this lifetime, the conclusion of its fantasy origins is further enforced. A traditionally trained Freudian therapist would most likely relate the story to childhood fantasies around toy soldiers, thus anchoring the origins of the story in actual events. A Jungian would concur in this but might add that the woods and the tree symbols suggest a symbolic regression to the realm of mother archetype. Both would nevertheless treat the imagery as psychological data valuable in understanding and unraveling certain personal complexes derived from this lifetime.

However, another approach to this piece of active imagination, derived from the past life therapy model, refines it into a much richer therapeutic drama, without losing any of Jung's essential priciple of staying with the image and imaginally living out the story.

The past life approach entails using a guide or therapist to focus the story and ask questions *as if* it were a literal lifetime event and not a fantasy, thus subjecting the story to the constraints of time, space, personal identity and history. This approach also acknowledges the limitations of the death experience and treats this too as a literal, bodily event when it occurs in the session. Much as these may sound like heavily weighted assumptions to use as the basis for leading questions, the finding of many thousands of regressions is that the psyche responds with great facility to the "as ifs" of such suggestions and frequently gives quite spontaneous and surprising historical data. Here is how the active imagination might typically be experienced as a past life memory:

Therapist (Th.): What are you doing?
Client (Cl.): I'm walking through the woods.
Th.: How are you dressed?
Cl.: Seems to be ragged clothes, a leather belt and pouch, and floppy hat, sort of medieval.
Th.: What kind of physique?
Cl.: I'm thick set, coarse, muscular, a peasant, about 30.
Th.: What happens in the woods?
Cl.: There are three soldiers coming out of the trees. Their swords are drawn.
Cl.: What are they doing?
Cl.: They're cutting my throat. Oh, I'm choking on my blood (coughs). I'm dying (convulses). I'm gone (body relaxes).
Th.: What are you aware of now?
Cl.: I'm, quite detached now. It's all over. I'm leaving.
Th.: Where do you go?
Cl.: I'm in a peaceful place above the earth. There are these beings with me. Very warm and comforting.
Th.: Are they human?
Cl.: No, not at all. They seem to be helpers. We communicate without talking. I don't seem to have a body now.

The dialogue is actually a composite, typical of many hundreds of past life sessions, but it differs in several important respects from the piece of unguided active imagination from which it developed. First, the story is now much more vivid; the imagery comes alive and forms a more psychologically authentic narrative. Second, the therapist's guiding assumptions of "as if" leads to a realistic death experience complete with choking and convulsions, which provides an emotional catharsis rather than a compensatory escape into a safe fantasy or memory. Third, the "as if" dialogue produces a distinction between two types of reality within the realm of the imagination. The embodied earthy reality of the peasant contrasts with the disembodied heavenly reality of the after-death state, where the subject easily distinguishes a different kind of presence from the soldiers. Whether these beings are called spirit guides or archetypal figures or angels, they clearly are not imaged as flesh and blood creatures like the soldiers.

This technique, then, expands the Jungian injunction to "stay with the image" by adding to it a metapsychological framework that allows more than one reality in which the individual's psychological complexes can be played out imaginally. Moreover, it includes the crucial archetypal rite of passage experience of the death transition from one reality to another. The other rite of passage between the two realities, is of course, birth; an example of this appears below.

Hypnotic inductions into past life scenarios

There are a number of effective hypnotic inductions that can be used to induce past life scenarios. Widely used are guided imagery protocols, which usually involve a fantasy journey leading to some kind of transitional image — a doorway, a bridge, a boat, a stairway, an elevator, a hot air balloon etc. — which signals to the unconscious a change of levels to another reality (for examples, see Reference 18). Sometimes this transition is made using an imaginary time line, or a calendar whose dates go back in time (this of course limits the past life experience to known historical eras, however).

Many hypnotherapists, used to practicing childhood regression, use the suggestion of going back through birth, to conception and 'earlier'. Some past life therapists standardly start with a birth regression before proceeding into past lives.[20] What is remarkable to anyone who uses these modalities is the way that the unconscious mind readily accepts these suggestions and produces detailed and often fully embodied images of past life characters and scenarios almost instantaneously. Coaching the subject to produce details is rarely necessary unless the scene recovered is one which entails a state of shock. In fact, most blocking of past life inductions is not due to the inability of the subject to access past life material but because a highly traumatic memory has been triggered which he or she resists reliving.

A much more direct induction to access past life scenarios involves the Gestalt or psycho-dramatic focusing of the therapeutic issue through phrases, images, or feeling relevant to the complex. This entails focusing on a highly charged issue in the client's current life situation, or possibly a traumatic scene in childhood, and extracting phrases or images that encapsulate the issue. For example:

> Therapist (Th.): Put words to those feelings you have about your life today.
> Client (Cl.): There's no one here for me. I always have to do everything alone.
> Th.: Repeat those words several times and let the unconscious take you to another lifetime when you first felt them.
> Cl.: There's no one there for me. There's no one here for me (several times). Where is everybody? They've all gone. What am I going to do?
> Th.: Where are you now?
> Cl.: I'm in this burnt out building. It's my home. The Indians! They took everyone (weeps).

This technique of repeating phrases can be found in the practice of Dianetics and is used effectively by many therapists who do not favor hypnosis.[20,28] Of course, this technique bears many resemblances to the hypnotherapy technique called the affect bridge.

Another highly effective and extremely swift induction into a past scenario which will inevitably be traumatic entails focusing on the kinesthetic awareness of a body pain, symptom or chronic postural pattern that epitomizes the client's presenting complaint. Here the therapist needs to listen for implicit images embedded in the description of the pain which will allow a transition to an imagined scene, via an "as if" suggestion.

> Therapist (Th.): What is this pain in your neck like?
> Client (Cl.): It's like a tight band around my neck, almost choking me.
> Th.: If it were made of something, this band, what would it be? Rope? Wood? Metal?
> Cl.: It's definitely metal. Its like a collar, and it's as if I'm being dragged by it. Oh help! They're dragging me, I'm a slave. I'm chained to all these other slaves. I'll never get away.

Past lives as psychodrama

> The play's the thing, wherein I'll catch the conscience
> of the King. Shakespeare, *Hamlet*, II, ii, 641

If we read the stage directions to any play, we find that everything is written in the present tense, grammatically speaking (e.g., "It is night. The old barn has a small lamp shining dimly above the door. The farmer and his son enter down stage. They are arguing fiercely"). In guiding a past life session, it is extremely helpful to follow this model by keeping the subject firmly in the present, having him recount the story as it happens, event by event, very much as if he or she were in the middle of a drama. Whenever the therapist poses a series of questions in any "past" tense, this acts as an unconscious trigger which can easily distance the subject from the events of the story so that imagery quickly loses its vividness.

Often during a past life session when a client is being moved forward in time, he or she will overshoot large sections of the story and will spontaneously begin describing the events in the past as over and finished. More often than not this indicates a strong resistance to reliving the painful core of the event. To counter this, the therapist needs to refocus in the present. For example:

> Therapist (Th.): Go forward to the next significant event.
> Client (Cl.): I'm living alone in the woods. The village ... it's all been destroyed. they came and ... killed everyone. (sadness in voice.)
> Th.: Go back to when you first find the village destroyed.
> Cl.: I see smoldering ruins ... bodies ... ugh! It's awful ... Oh no, no ... (sobs) ... It's my wife! (deep sobbing).

Sometimes the opposite resistance occurs; the subject does not want to go forward in time because the unconscious mind is already anticipating painful scenes. In this case, it is common for an earlier scene to be dragged out moment by moment, almost in slow motion, so that the subject appears frozen in time. To counter this kind of blocking, it is helpful to use phrases with the present tense. For example, "What do you find when you go upstairs?" or "What happens when you do go into battle?"

An even more subtle linguistic way of dissolving this kind of block is used by Morris Netherton. This is the use of a conditional tense:

> Therapist (Th.): What happened now?
> Client (Cl.): I don't know. I don't want to go to the door.
> Th.: What would happen if you did?
> Cl.: There would be men there.
> Th.: What would they do?
> Cl.: (trembling) They would beat me up and drag me off for interrogation.
> Th.: So how do they drag you off?
> Cl.: I'm kicking and struggling. They've hit me over the head. It's a black van. They're Gestapo. Oh, no, no!

'How?' questions are among the most valuable for bringing the zoom lens right in close to the traumatic event. In fact, I have noticed that therapists in training will sometimes avoid these questions themselves if a particularly gruesome scene of torture or mutilation is involved. Usually this avoidance is because some past life trauma of their own is unresolved on these issues. Nevertheless, in order for a trauma of this nature to be fully released at a psychosomatic level, the exact details have to be elicited by the therapist with all the precision of a surgeon removing shrapnel from the tissue of a bomb victim.

To illustrate this difficult aspect of work, I will cite a case from my practice in which a young woman did actually remember dying in a bomb explosion. The physical feature that was most prominent in her current life when she came for therapy was that she was suffering from lupus, which caused arthritis-like pains in the joints of her arms and legs. In the past life session, she re-lived the life of a young anarchist in Czarist Russia at the turn of the century. The crucial scene was as follows:

> Therapist (Th.): What are you doing now?
> Client (Cl.): We're carrying bombs, They're for those bastards (soldiers who killed my sister).
> Th.: Go forward and tell me what happens.
> Cl.: It's all black. I'm not in my body.
> Th.: Go back and describe to me how you die.
> Cl.: I'm looking down from outside my body. Oh my God! It has no arms and legs. There's been an explosion. It's still moving.

Th.: Go back inside your body and tell me exactly how it feels.
Cl.: I'm dying, lying here on the street. The pain is terrible. No arms, no legs ... (cries) ... Now I'm dead, No more movement. I'm leaving the body.
Th.: As you leave, be aware that you don't have to carry that pain anymore.

Similiar to most victims of explosions, the young anarchist had gone out of his body, even thought he was not yet dead. The death agony was unfinished and was recorded in the imaginal body memory of the anarchist life. It would seem that this memory had been imprinted on the young woman's body in this lifetime as part of the lupus symptom of pain in her joints. (See Reference 29 for the theory of subtle body imprints from past lives.) For her, letting go of the physical memories also entailed letting go of the vengeful feelings she (he) had carried as the young anarchist, which had symbolically turned against her as "explosive" rage. What is remarkable is that after this one session all the arthritis-like symptoms disappeared. Her doctor, who was present at the session, attests that the symptoms did not return, over two years later.

Catharsis, resistance, and the subtle body

The examples we have just cited illustrate vividly the third basic principle that is essential, in my experience, for effective cathartic working through in past life therapy: the subject must fully re-experience the bodily sensations of the past life trauma for emotional and energetic release to be complete.

If these bodily sensations and their concomitant emotions are not fully experienced, the psychological complex seeking to express itself will remain lodged in the body, as it were. No amount of methodical understanding of the meaning, symbolic content, or "karmic" ramifications of the experience will help unless this bodily imagery is allowed to surface as well .

The reverse is also true: If the physical and emotional levels of the trauma are released without a full understanding of their meaning, in whatever framework the subject is open to (psychological, karmic, spiritual), then the subject will tend to remain stuck in a meaningless repetition of the emotions of the past life scenario; whatever psychosomatic symptoms existed will continue. In the case of the lupus sufferer just cited, it was just as essential for her to understand the symbolic meaning of the explosion (as rage that had backfired against her in that lifetime) as it was for her to re-experience the death.

Being aware of one's previous life though the subtle body is thus a further extension of the Jungian precept to "stay with the image." Only now it may be expressed as "stay in your body" with the dual meaning of

1. staying in the subtle body of the *other* lifetime
2. being aware of *this* lifetime's body sensations as you remember the other life

In other words, therapy has to be sensitive to this overlay as the cause of psychosomatic symptoms. Bringing the body image into a past life scenario makes the unconscious imprinting of the subtle body less concrete and frees up libido (or orgone energy, or chi, or prana) for creative and spiritual purposes. Thus in our sessions we move from the literal to the symbolic to its release in the present. Current backache becomes a past life "broken back," which leads to a discovery of new impetus for life. Current migraine headaches become a past life "head injury," which leads to a freeing from burdensome and painful thoughts.

Not being in the body is another version of the schizoid defense of distancing in time we described earlier. Just as in the examples given, where the subject had to be gently brought back or forward to the crucial existential moment of the trauma, so with certain experiences the subject must be brought fully into the body. Sometimes it is even necessary to exaggerate the imaginal psychodrama by urging deep breathing by the client, or by applying massage or some kind of physical pressure to appropriate pressure points on the client's body.

As an example of this, we may cite the case of young woman who described a previous life when, as a twelve year old girl, she had been killed in a Nazi gas chamber. Her account in her first session of her deportation to a concentration camp and subsequent death, though detailed, was extremely flat, detached, without catharsis. Painful as it was, we decide to re-run the memory, this time refocusing both dramatically and physically:

> Therapist (Th.): Where are you now?
> Client (Cl.): We're in a line outside a building. I'm no longer with my mother.
> Th.: What exactly are you doing?
> Cl.: I'm holding the hand of this older woman.
> Th.: How do you feel?
> Cl.: Terrible!
> Th.: Do you cry?
> Cl.: No, I can't.
> Th.: All right. Then breathe very deeply and let any feelings you may be holding back come to the surface (coaches breathing).
> Cl.: (breathing deeply) I don't want to go in there (trembles, heaves).
> Th.: Say that louder.
> Cl.: *I don't want to go in there* (sobs loudly).

From then on a flood of emotion emerged and she described in detail the gassing: how it tasted, smelled, and which parts of her body it affected. For several minutes she went though the convulsions of choking, vomiting, and doubling up as she re-lived her death.

By the end of the session she had released so much fear, grief, despair and physical pain, that her chest had opened up to a much fuller pattern of breathing, similar to the releases experienced in Reichian therapy and re-birthing. Later she reported that a deep-seated depression, which seemed to be with her most of her life, was gone and that her breathing pattern was permanently changed.

In her case there were no particular indications in her appearance of these bodily blocks. Her breathing had been shallow initially, it was true, but not exceptionally shallow, so the chief clue to her block was the lack of affect in her memory. In other cases the body image advertises "trauma" much more loudly so to speak, and then more direct intervention may be appropriate.

This was true of a 34 year-old female painter who sought out therapy reciting a confused bag of complaints about her marriage, about the bad feelings she had about her mother (from whom she had moved away); she also mentioned the notion that it was all connected to a past life fragment she had glimpsed as a painter in Holland. As she told her story, I was struck by how rigid and tense her shoulders were. It was as though they were held two or three inches higher than necessary.

During the relaxation part of my induction procedure she had great difficulty in letting go of her shoulder muscles, so I offered to massage her neck and shoulders. When she agreed, I worked a little on her very tight trapezius muscle and her neck. Very soon she slipped into a male life as in impoverished Dutch painter during the 17th century. The painter had a wife and a very young baby, whom he could barely support.

In his obsession with finishing a certain painting, he severely neglected both wife and baby, even when the baby became sick. To his horror the baby grew worse and died, and his embittered wife deserted him. The key scene in our work was as follows:

> Therapist (Th.): Where are you now?
> Client (Cl.): I'm wandering along the canals. I can't find my wife. She's left me for good.
> Th.: Where do you go now?
> Cl.: I think, back to the house. Oh, no! I don't want to go back there. (Her shoulders begin to tense up very noticeably).
> Th.: Breath deeply and go back to the house and see what happens. (At this point, the young woman client shot up from lying on the couch to a sitting position. She grabbed her neck and began to scream.)
> Th.: What has happened?
> Cl.: Oh God! I hanged myself. (Sobs deeply).

For a short while we worked on letting go of the death experience and the emotions connected with the loss of wife and child. But this was not all. When asked to move forward, she spontaneously found herself re-experiencing her birth in this current life, with the umbilical cord wrapped around her neck! Full understanding came moments later when, as the newborn baby, she looked up at her mother, having survived this second trauma.

Cl.: I know why I'm here
Th.: Why are you here?
Cl.: To be close to my mother. (sobs) I know who she is now.
Th.: Tell me who she is.
Cl.: She's the baby who died (in the Dutch lifetime). I see that I've been trying to make it up to her all these years.

What is remarkable about this exceptionally condensed session is the way in which all the guilt about the neglect and the death of the baby had been lodged, as an imaginal imprint in her neck and shoulders, at the moment of the Dutch painter's remorseful suicide.

All her feelings about the Dutch baby and her current mother were reinforced in the birth trauma and carried in the young woman's body language to the present day. They had remained locked in her neck and shoulders. She had continued to punish herself unconsciously and had not been able to let go of feeling responsible for her mother. In subsequent sessions she could release this burden. She felt enormous pressure taken off her marriage, to say nothing of her shoulders, which had by then noticeably dropped a couple of inches.

Past life bodywork

Of course, not every client's body language speaks so loudly or so urgently, but almost any part of the body where there is chronic or recurrent pain may harbor the image of a past life trauma that can be effectively worked with. The well-known movement therapist, Anna Halpern, says that "every part of the body has a story to tell," perfectly summarizing the principle we have been illustrating.

How the therapist reaches the story, buried as it is in the body's unconscious fantasies, will vary according to what tools and training he or she brings to a past life session. We have seen how verbal cues can elicit the story, as can breathing and massage. It is noticeable, too, how more and more people sensitive to the past life dimension of the psyche are reporting fragments of past lives during Rolfing massage, primal therapy, and other forms of body work.[29]

Yet it must be stated clearly that any bodywork of this sort is only a means to eliciting a story, a story which belongs to the imaginal body. Altering body tissues cannot be an end in itself from the perspective of past life therapy; moreover, it is doomed to only limited success if the psyche is ignored. When a person complains of persistent back pain, the aim of a massage would be to allow a clear image of that pain to emerge as a key to an imaginal drama involving that location of the body in another lifetime. The therapist's task is to pursue the story in the understanding, confirmed by more and more reports, that it is the re-living of the story in all its physical details, psychological drama, and human pathos that really heals.

References

1. Bernstein, Morey, *The Search for Bridey Murphy*, Doubleday, New York, 1965.
2. Coward, Harold, *Jung and Eastern Thought*, SUNY Press, Albany, New York, 1985.
3. Dethlefsen, Thorwald, *Voices from Other Lives*, Evans, New York, 1978.
4. Dethlefsen, Thorwald, *The Challenge of Fate*, Coventure, Boston, 1984.
5. Fiore, Edith, *You Have Been Here Before*, Ballantine, NY, 1969.
6. Grant, Joan and Kelsey, Denys, *Many Lifetimes*, Pocket Books, New York, 1969.
7. Grof, Stanislav, *Beyond the Brain*, SUNY Press, Albany, NY, 1984.
8. Head, Joseph and Sylvia Cranston, Eds., *Reincarnation: the phoenix fire mystery*, Warner Books, New York, 1979.
9. Hubbard, L. Ron, *Have You Lived Before This Life?*, The Church of Scientology, Los Angeles, 1958.
10. Jung, C.G., On the psychology and pathology of so-called occult phenomena, in *Psychiatric Studies*, Coll. Works, 1, Princeton University Press, Princeton, NJ, 1957.
11. Jung, C.G., *The Structure and Dynamics of the Psyche*, Coll. Works, Vol. 8, Princeton University Press, Princeton, NJ, 1960, 22.
12. Jung, C.G., *The Practice of Psychotherapy*, Coll. Works, 16, Princeton University Press, Princeton, New Jersey, 1966.
13. Jung, C.G., *Memories, Dreams, Reflections*, Ed. Jaffe, Random House, New York, 1963.
14. Kardec, A., *The Spirit's Book*, Brotherhood of Life, Albuquerque, NM, 1989, (first published: Paris, 1857).
15. Kelsey, Denys and Joan Grant, *Many Lifetimes*, Doubleday, New York, 1967.
16. Langley, Noel, *Edgar Cayce on Reincarnation*, Warner, New York, 1967.
17. Lewis, James R. and J. Gordon Melton, *Perspectives on the New Age*, SUNY Press, New York, 1992.
18. Lucas, Winafred, *Regression Therapy: a handbook for professionals*, Deep Forest Press, Crest Park, CA, 1993.
19. McGregor, Geddes, *Reincarnation in Christianity*, Theosophical Pub., Wheaton, Illinois, 1978.
20. Netherton, Morris, and Shiffren, Nancy, *Past Lives Therapy*, William Morrow New York, 1978.
21. Rochas, Albert de, *Les vies successives*, Charcornal, Paris, 1911.
22. Rogo, D. Scott, *The Search for Yesterday*, Prentice-Hall, NJ, 1985.
23. Rossi, Ernest and David Cheek, *Mind Body Therapy*, Norton, New York, 1988.
24. Ten Dam, Hans, *Deep Healing: the methodology of past-life therapy*, Amsterdam, 1989.
25. Wambach, Helen, *Reliving Past Lives*, Bantam, New York, 1978.
26. Watkins, Mary, *Waking Dreams*, Gordon & Beach, New York, 1976.
27. Waveren, Erlo van, *Pilgrimage to the Rebirth*, Weiser, New York, 1978.
28. Woolger, Roger J., *Other Lives, Other Selves*, Doubleday, New York, 1987.
29. Woolger, Roger J., Aspects of Past Life Bodywork: understanding subtle energy fields, in *J. Regression Therapy*, II, 1, 2, Riverside, California, 1987.

For professional training and resources:

Woolger Training Seminars
1365B Bear Mountain Drive
Boulder, CO 80303
(303) 554-8300
www.woolger.com/regression

Association of Past-Life Research and Therapy
PO Box 20151
Riverside, CA 92516
(909) 784-1570

For further study:

Lucas, Winafred, *Regression Therapy: A Handbook for Professionals*, 2 vols., Deep Forest Press, Crest Park, CA, 1993.

chapter ten

Prenatal and perinatal hypnotherapy

David Chamberlain

Historical background

During the summer of 1974, I took my first training course in Clinical Applications of Hypnosis and was taught a rapid method of induction gleaned from techniques of Dave Elman.[1] I saw hypnotherapy as a logical system which treated symptoms by activating memories of seminal experiences. Then we worked to create understanding of the issues involved and chose alternative behaviors and feelings. I was repeatedly surprised by the narrative recall of traumatic incidents, some of them far in the past, including intrauterine and birth experiences.

At the time, I knew little of the history of primal work, utilizing hypnosis or any other means, and I was too ignorant to ask clients to go back to womb or birth events to find the roots of a problem. Clients simply took me there and described their experiences to me, often leaving both of us equally puzzled. When I was shown the publications of David Cheek, obstetrician and hypnosis pioneer, detailing accurate recall of head and shoulder sequences at birth[2] as well as maladjustment patterns related to imprinting at birth,[3] I was tremendously encouraged. We became friends and colleagues over the next twenty years before his death in 1996.

What struck me about these early narratives was the precocious, apparently innate, and unpredicted qualities of feeling, perception, and cognition that were coming "out of the mouths of babes." Because pre- and perinatal feeling, perception, and cognition were considered impossible within the then current paradigm of developmental psychology, practitioners usually ended up explaining such memories as fantasies and projections. Psychologists supposed clients were using adult vocabulary and semantics to describe feelings, perceptions, and thoughts which could not possibly have existed before larynx, tongue, and airways could form adult language.

Professionals quarreled about the more fundamental issue of whether *any* thought or memory could be laid down during the prenatal or perinatal era. I learned that this debate carried all the way back to Sigmund Freud's and Otto Rank's time and attitudes and beliefs were little changed since then. When I spoke of birth memories, my psychology colleagues reminded me that there was insufficient myelination (fatty sheathing around nerve pathways) to permit cognitive activity in newborns. This scientific sounding view was later seen as irrelevant, since myelination is not complete until adolescence, and it mainly effects the *speed* of nerve transmission which is not a significant factor in the tiny body of an infant.

Another scientific prejudice was skepticism regarding anecdotal data, i.e., data from personal experience, and clinical data from clients in therapy. Most scientists believed authoritative knowledge could *only* be gained from physiological or experimental research, yet this research was lagging far behind what people were discovering for themselves. Although public perceptions of mental or psychic possibilities have been powerfully affected by thousands of personal reports, scientific resistance to this type of evidence has remained almost unchanged. This helps to explain why no serious scientific attention was paid to the first published reports in 1981[4] that children were sharing spontaneous memories of birth as they were first learning to speak. This *prima facie* evidence made not a dent on psychological theories of memory, including the specious belief in "infantile amnesia" which held on stubbornly until its demise in the 1990s.[5]

As I pursued my clinical work and listened to what eventually became hundreds of narrative reports regarding womb and birth memories, I began a long term study of everything known about the capabilities of infants. This new field of research, beginning in the late 1970s, expanded exponentially in the 80s and 90s. I published reviews of these findings in papers[6] and in my book, *The Mind of Your Newborn Baby*,[7] I was able to set birth memory in this larger context of empirical information.

Transpersonal adventures

Prenatal and perinatal memories are transpersonal in transcending all the expected boundaries of consciousness during intrauterine time and birth, especially memory, learning, sensation, emotion, perception, thought, dreaming, out-of-body experience, near-death experience, clairvoyance, and telepathy. *None* of these phenomena of consciousness were anticipated in the materialistic paradigm of 20th century developmental psychology. In fact they were rejected as impossible because they did not fit the standard paradigm. Nevertheless, individuals demonstrated these capacities.

In my experience, clients, regardless of their age at the time of memory formation, always presented the full spectrum of consciousness that I now regard as *normative*. They always possessed a sense of self, an awareness of the environment, an interest in relationships, and always appeared to be trying to grasp the meaning of things, or otherwise coping with their experiences. This is not to say that they always displayed perfect understanding. In therapeutic work, distortions in thinking became obvious and often required reframing in order to escape the grip of fears, anxieties, and compulsive behavior patterns.

The view of life presented by babies at birth is an intriguing and mystical one of complete persons in little bodies knowing many things: they are frustrated that they cannot yet make their bodies work the way they'd like; they know what they need and whom they can trust; they evaluate the motivations of doctors; they perceive the psychological flaws in standard medical births; they point out virtues or weaknesses of parents; and they recognize the special needs of their siblings.

Examples from my practice

In private practice as a psychologist, I dealt with many patients suffering from depression, fear and anxieties. As a starting point, I suggested to clients that these symptoms might be learned responses associated with past experiences, asking them whether they had any conscious memories or hunches about what those experiences could have been. This approach was very productive, and it seemed to make them feel better right away — I suppose because their own theories about what was wrong with them were much worse. Of course, sometimes, no conscious memories came to their minds, so I offered hypnotherapy as a way of exploring deeper in their memories to see what they might have forgotten. Sometimes, clients responded to my suggestion by spontaneously entering trance as they began contemplating the past for clues to their condition. Others needed only the slightest permission; they were already getting impressions or unconsciously moving parts of their body before I got very far into my induction. I came to understand that such clients were more ready to do the necessary work than I was. The following are examples of transpersonal phenomena which appeared as we were seeking the origin of a symptom.

Maxine was allergic to confusion and said that she hated her mother "from day one." After using an induction drawn from Elman including a couple of exercises in specific amnesia, this business woman in her midforties responded to the suggestion to remember "day one" and her first encounter with her mother. Inside, all was peaceful, she said, but as soon as she came out, confusion reigned. Her mother was at the center of it, first by doing a lot of yelling, then by talking constantly and making critical and contradictory remarks to the baby. Maxine had no trouble reporting on words spoken at the time. Everyone present had greeted her as a girl but mother announced to father that she was a boy, a cause of consternation. "I didn't know what to think" she said. Reacting to my questions about her sense of identity in utero, she explained she did not think in terms of male or female but said "I knew I was born of God." "I knew God was sending me, was making me," she said. She had keen perceptions about the family and knew her brother and father liked her, as did the nurse and doctor, but mother was in a different category. Mother was strange, contradictory, very emotional, and she felt rejected by her. "Why are you here? I don't know how to take care of you. You're no good," said mother. The world was a confusing place; Maxine said, "It was hard for me to adjust to this world."

In emergencies, newborns recalling birth sometimes show unexpected concern, objectivity, and compassion. In a hectic crisis some babies remain cool, know they are safe and try to reassure their helpers that all will be well. Kate was a woman in her thirties who presented with fear of suffocation and a persistent feeling of unworthiness to be in a close relationship. After a brief induction with the same features as above, Kate began to abreact, recalling first a fear of suffocation provoked during anesthesia for a childhood tonsillectomy. Then, responding to my suggestion that she could go further back to when she first experienced suffocation, she recalled in great detail a life and death struggle at her birth. Her story takes us into an unimagined world of moral dilemmas, decisions, thoughts, and feelings. She realized the womb had filled with blood and she feared that if she came out, her mother might die. With agonizing sobs she said, "If I come out and she dies, she'll never know how much I love her! I want to know her. She talked to me a lot before I was born but nobody else knew because they'd think it was silly. I felt like I was going to drown, and I knew I wasn't supposed to … Ohhh, they just don't understand what's happening." As her lengthy abreaction unfolded, the origin of her sense of guilt and unworthiness seemed definitely set in the matrix of nearly killing the mother she loved, just by being born.

During an extended resuscitation period after delivery, Kate seemed completely familiar with the thoughts, emotions, and actions of the attending doctor and nurse. "The nurse wants the doctor to just stop because she thinks I'm dead! The doctor just told her to shut up … They're not going to stop! It feels like my body's shriveling up. That's why the nurse keeps saying, 'She's dead.' She wants to go home. They've been there all night…."

Stewart, a young, conscientious professional, had a severe case of procrastination. As he recalled the origin of his procrastination in trance, he found himself at birth. Although born with a clear sense of self, his narrative recall showed how severely his sense of identity was tested (and was powerfully programmed) by labels the doctor hurled at him in the delivery room. Talking to the mother, the doctor called him a "difficult kid … not like regular children … and probably would be late for everything." He says, "Mrs. E., you have a stubborn child … not quite normal. They're supposed to drop their hands, and he's not." You can hear Stewart struggling to maintain his identity, "He's rough! His words are coarse, not gentle at all … He was saying to mother that I was going to be a difficult kid. I'm not, but he said I was, and everybody was in agreement. Nobody was taking my side. I wanted to say, 'No, I'm not!' But they wouldn't listen."

Babies sometimes explicitly express a metaphysical orientation. Exploring her birth in trance, Linda understood what she "had" to do after birth and was reluctant to do it: "I have to put myself in that baby body," she said. She had the insight that when she was born, she felt "wise" and knew a lot, but by the time she was three, she had become a conventional child fitting into the role expected of her. She became "that dumb little kid" everybody thought she should be, and had to grow up to become wise again. Nan, whose first day after birth was full of disappointments, began to weep, saying "Perhaps the whole thing was a mistake. I wanted to go back." (She was sure her mother was going to smother her!)

Marybeth had a very different experience from Nan. She says of her feelings at birth: "I felt warm, safe, content, a self-assured child, but very wise, a wise person in a child's body."

Emily says of her father's awkwardness in first meeting her after her birth, "He doesn't know I'm a person; I'm a *thing* called a baby. He's saying, 'That's all the babies; this one was hard enough!' I didn't think I was that hard ... I don't think I like these people ... They give me a headache ... They don't think I'm a person! I *know* I am."

All birth reports reveal an active mind, but few contain such forthright declarations of mind as this one by my client, Deborah, looking back at her experience with people in the delivery room. "I felt I knew a lot — I really did. I thought I was pretty intelligent. I never thought about being a person, just a mind. And so when the situation was forced on me, I didn't like it too much. I saw all these people acting real crazy. That's when I thought I really had a more intelligent mind, because I knew what the situation was with me, and they didn't seem to. They seemed to ignore me. They were doing things *to* me, to the *outside* of me. But they acted like that's all there was. When I tried to tell them things, they just wouldn't listen, like that noise wasn't really anything. It didn't sound too impressive, but it was all I had. I just really felt like I was more intelligent than they were."

Judging from reported womb and birth memories, babies may be capable of the same variety of altered states of consciousness that adults experience: being out-of-body, near-death, observing the death of a twin in utero, and traveling to realms of sublime love and limitless knowing. Such reports typically come as a surprise and often are not consciously understood, suggesting that these states are unfamiliar and need further interpretation. Laura, having what I would identify as an out-of-body experience in the hospital nursery, said: "I feel weightless, floating. Nobody knows I'm there; they can't even see me. I keep looking through the nursery window; it's weird. I can't be on both sides of the window! I'm looking at the baby; it's me."

Jeannette, at 41, sought hypnotherapy for her life long insomnia. Falling asleep often triggered a panic attack that woke her up with her heart pounding. In hypnosis, she recalled a near-death experience in the womb, caused by acidic chemicals introduced by her mother at the insistence of her drunken father! In childhood, she said, she had always feared her father and never knew why. During her uterine crisis her heart was beating very hard. "My body was filled up with my heart beating faster and faster until it killed me," she said. She described the sensations as "searing." When her heart raced in the night, she was afraid to sleep because she associated this racing heartbeat with death. "I'm afraid I'll slip back into death. I believe I need high-powered, adrenalized action to stay alive."

A related problem for Jeanette was nightmares containing death scenes and body parts. In hypnosis she recalled her anguish and terror in the womb. She wanted to crawl into a dark hole and hide. "It's hard to breathe. I want out. I want to dig my eyes out! I'm so uncomfortable. Everything seems wrong ... There's nothing here to help me. I need help! I'm really alone, so lonely! There's no way of fixing it! I don't want to be alone. It doesn't seem right to be alone." What Jeanette discovered was that the attempted abortion in which she had nearly died had killed her twin sister. She was then haunted by the experience of observing her sister's gradual disintegration. She explained, "the worst part was seeing her disintegrate into parts ... This is why I wanted to scratch my eyes out." One of her worst fears was "to stare death in the face," one of the recurring themes in her nightmares.

For Jeanette, a further consequence of these events in utero was a phobic response to all babies and a persistent jealousy of twins. As a mature woman she had no urge to have children; indeed, she had no confidence that she could "create a good womb environment" in which a baby could survive. To her, babies seemed "spooky." "When I see a baby, I see violence being done to it. It gives me a wild feeling of thrashing and fighting," she said. "I feared some evil would overtake them and that they might disintegrate."

Before connecting these terrors with her experiences in the womb, which we were able to do together in hypnosis, they had made no sense to her; they simply haunted her and left her swimming in anxiety. After hypnotherapy she had a new lease on life, began to sleep normally, could remain calm in critical situations, and even considered having a child of her own. Her fear of death was finally resolved after returning to her own death experience in hypnosis; she discovered that her death had involved visiting a luminous realm of safety and love where all knowledge was immediately available to her. This was an astonishing new idea of death.

Changing paradigms

The complex consciousness of babies revealed in hypnotherapy became for me a window for seeing the complexities and potentialities of all human consciousness. Babies taught me that age was not a requirement for consciousness. Indeed, consciousness was not a developmental trait, but an innate endowment of human persons. Increasingly, prenatal research reveals more sentience than can be explained by old theories of neurological development.[8]

This counter-cultural view challenges the entrenched, materialistic paradigm of 20th century psychology and medicine which defines persons as matter, especially brain matter. If there is no brain matter, then there can be no person, no cognition, and no consciousness. On this faulty premise, all discoveries of prenatal or perinatal consciousness have been discounted or denied since inadequate brain resources would make them impossible. Psychologists, neonatologists, and obstetricians manage to hold onto this 19th century view of babies by ignoring the findings about consciousness in near-death research,[9] particularly the verified observations made while out-of-body (and brain), the empirical confirmations of past life memory, and the whole range of psychic phenomena, including evidence of the telepathy between mothers and babies.[10] Children who are just learning to talk are as likely to have spontaneous past life recall as they are to have birth and womb recall.[11]

Although hypnosis has often been the handmaiden of consciousness, revealing the inner workings of the mind and spirit, its contributions have been stubbornly resisted in psychiatry, in psychology, in the branches of medicine which deal with babies, and even in professional hypnosis societies. I believe much of this skepticism is the direct result of medical training which equates brain and person. This restricted paradigm can no longer explain the evidence which is flooding in from anecdotal, clinical, and research sources.

The leaders of American psychology made a pragmatic decision at the beginning of the century to exclude studies of consciousness because consciousness was more philosophy than science, and psychology was determined to be scientific. It has taken the better part of the century for psychology to regain its humanistic and its transpersonal agenda.

In obstetrics and psychology, ultrasound technology is overturning a century of pet theories of development. As systematic observations of fetal behavior accumulate, it is already becoming apparent that babies hear before they have ears, see before they have eyes, move gracefully and spontaneously before they have much brain, communicate telepathically with their mothers and fathers before they have language, move in and out of the body, carry past life memories, make decisions and begin to shape their lives around their intrauterine experiences. Ultrasound is revealing the heretofore secret life of twins and their unimagined social relationships beginning at only 20 weeks after conception.[12] Stories are circulating of babies attacking amniocentesis needles, which typically enter the womb around 16 weeks from conception, while parents and professionals watch it all happen on the ultrasound monitor. To explain these phenomena, a much larger paradigm is needed, one that embraces the whole spectrum of consciousness.

Transpersonal paths converge

While I was having my adventures in transpersonal hypnotherapy, I was continually reminded that there were other roads to prenatal realms of consciousness. A friend of mine who presided over a college of massage reported that the mere lifting of an arm would periodically result in birth abreactions in the midst of a Swedish massage. In England and the United States, psychiatrists using LSD in controlled experiments discovered that people could access their womb and birth traumas (among other transpersonal phenomena), and when LSD was no longer legal, they found it possible to achieve the same effects by use of movement and music. Others found a different route via yogic breathing, fantasy procedures, free-association, dreams, or therapeutic art. Recently, people have been reporting that working with specific parts of the feet is likely to provoke memories of the prenatal period. My own experience has been with using hypnosis as "the royal road to the unconscious."

Over these last two decades, the validity of hypnosis itself has been continually debated and tested, as theories compete and evolve. I have, of course, noted that some people are more suggestible than others, and that the circumstances or conditions can make a difference in their responsiveness to hypnosis. "Depth" of hypnosis has not proved to be necessary, nor have special efforts or techniques been required for work in the prenatal period. Some people are so "ready" to work that they arrive at an early trauma while I am just beginning the induction process. This has reinforced the idea that hypnosis, or trance, is a natural phenomenon that occurs spontaneously in everyday life. Memories of past trauma, though apparently forgotten, can be brought to the surface by current conditions. That they are not truly forgotten is coherent with recent theories of infant memory as a way of learning from and incorporating experience. Memory as the foundation under all new experiences is never lost, although it may slip from conscious recall and need to be refreshed.[13]

Under trance conditions, life circumstances may trigger flashbacks in adults, and children may act out their memories in play. Invariably, I find that my new clients have been having spontaneous flashbacks without realizing it. Memories of unresolved trauma were literally knocking at the door. I immediately encourage them to respect these revelations while we proceed to use hypnosis as a more orderly means of discovery.

Summary

When I began using hypnotherapy as a tool in my psychology practice in 1974, prenatal and perinatal memories were considered an impossible feat for infant brains and were labeled fantasies. This general view has not changed much in almost a quarter century of medicine and psychology. Then, as now, a minority of practitioners were fascinated by these early memories, struggled to understand them, and, even if they couldn't accept them as "real," they put such material to constructive clinical use since it was important to their clients. Others turned to rejection and ridicule, setting aside evidence in favor of the prevailing dogma.

I attribute this scientific "failure to progress" to the resilience of an outdated paradigm of human nature which defines persons *only* as matter — particularly as brain matter. Transpersonal phenomena plainly overflow the banks of this old paradigm and suggest a larger truth, not yet fully articulated, of mind and soul as *consciousness*. Uncovering the mind/soul of infants through hypnotherapy has been a priceless adventure for me, as well as a gateway to understanding the larger issues of human consciousness. As we continue to discover babies for who they are, knowledge of infant consciousness will play a strong part in convincing the world, including the academic world, to shift to a new paradigm of human consciousness that goes far beyond the artificial and material boundaries we have previously set for it.

References

1. Elman, D., *Hypnotherapy*, Westwood Publishing, Glendale, CA, 1970.
2. Cheek, D.B., Sequential head and shoulder movements appearing with age regression in hypnosis to birth, *Am. J. Clinical Hypnosis*, 16(4), 261–266, 1974.
3. Cheek, D.B., Maladjustment patterns apparently related to imprinting at birth, *Am. J. Clinical Hypnosis*, 18(2), 75–82, 1975.
4. Matthison, L.A., Does your child remember? *Mothering*, 21, Fall, 103–107, 1981.
5. Bauer, P.J., What do infants recall of their lives? Memory for specific events by one- to two-year olds. *American Psychologist*, 51(1), 29–41, 1996, Rovee-Collier, C., Shifting the focus from what to why. *Infant Behavior and Development*, 19, 385–400, 1996.
6. Chamberlain, D.B., The cognitive newborn: A scientific update. *Br. J. of Psychotherapy*, 4(1), 30-71, 1987; Chamberlain, D.B., Babies are not what we thought: Call for a new paradigm. *International J. Prenatal and Perinatal Studies*. 4(3/4), 161–177, 1992.
7. Chamberlain, D.B., *The Mind of Your Newborn Baby*, 3rd ed., North Atlantic Books, Berkeley, CA, 1998.
8. Chamberlain, D.B., The sentient prenate: What every parent should know, *Pre- and Perinatal Psychol. J.*, 9(1), 9–31, 1994.
9. Ring, K., *Life at death: A scientific investigation of the near-death experience*, Coward, Mc Cann and Goehegan, New York, 1980.
10. Cheek, D.B., Prenatal and perinatal imprints: apparent prenatal consciousness as revealed by hypnosis, *Pre- and Perinatal Psychology J.*, 1(2), 97–110, 1986; Cheek, D.B., Are telepathy, clairvoyance and "hearing" possible in utero? Suggestive evidence as revealed during hypnotic age-regression studies of prenatal memory, *Pre- and Perinatal Psychology J.*, 7(2), 125–137, 1992.
11. Stevenson, I., Children who remember past lives: A question of reincarnation, University Press of Virginia, Charlottesville, VA, 1987.
12. Piontelli, A., *From fetus to child: An observational and psychoanalytic study.*, Tavistock/Routledge, London and New York, 1992.
13. Rovee-Collier, C., Shifting the focus from what to why, *Infant Behavior and Development*, 19, 385–400, 1996.

For further study:

Association for Pre- and Perinatal Psychology and Health
340 Colony Road
Geyservillle, CA 95441
(707) 857-4041 (phone)
(707) 857-4042 (fax)
Email: apppah@aol.com
Web Site: http://www.birthpsychology.com

The Journal of Prenatal and Perinatal Psychology and Health has been published quarterly since 1986. For more information, contact the Association office or web site above.

chapter eleven

Spirit Releasement Therapy

Joseph Wicker

Introduction

Spirit Releasement Therapy was developed by Dr. William Baldwin who originally called this work Clinical Depossession. Although others have done this work extensively over the years, especially therapists associated with Past Life Therapy work, Dr. Baldwin has done more than anyone to organize, teach, and promote this type of therapy during recent years. His technique manual, entitled *Spirit Releasement Therapy*,[2] is in its second edition, and is a key source of information for any qualified therapist interested in this work.

Spirit Releasement Therapy is considered by some therapists as a therapy within itself, while others consider it to be more properly classified as a therapeutic technique. For the purposes of this chapter, it will be considered as a therapeutic technique to be used in the context of an ongoing therapeutic relationship. This is particularly important since differential diagnosis conducted by a trained mental health professional is crucial in doing this work. Therefore, throughout this chapter, Spirit Releasement Therapy (SRT) will be used to refer to this therapeutic technique.

The word *spirit* as used in this context refers to a wide range of spirits or entities that can attach to or influence the human energy field. Often called *attached entities* in the literature, these entities are generally broadly classified as either deceased, earthbound, human spirits, or as other discarnate entities. As noted above, it is crucial for the therapist doing this type of work to be educated and trained in doing differential diagnosis since these types of entities need to be differentiated from ego states or subpersonalities, personality fragments, alter personalities in someone with Dissociative Identity Disorder, pastlife memories or personalities, spirit guides, etc. These entities also need to be differentiated from psychotic material such as delusions and hallucinations.

Entities that are earthbound human spirits are spirits which for one reason or another (for example, confused about being dead or afraid to go on to the Light) have remained on the earth plane and have attached to some other person's energy field. Discarnate entities are various types of entities that have never manifested in human form but can operate on the earth plane. These include spirit guides, angels, demons or dark entities of various sorts, walk-ins, exterterrestial entities, etc.

Obviously, such material will stretch or overstep the bounds of some therapists' credulity. It is essential that professionals who do this type of work have a working knowledge of metaphysics, spirituality, and nonphysical levels of reality. Otherwise much of the material may be foreign and open to misinterpretation. Whether these entities are real in the metaphysical sense and/or real in the phenomenal sense as part of the patient's experiential reality is beyond the scope of this chapter and at some level is probably a nonsensical query. That this material is dealt with in an appropriate and therapeutic manner that helps to alleviate the patient's symptoms and promote their healing and ability to function effectively in life is what is of paramount importance.

Spirit Releasement Therapy as a therapeutic technique is utilized with the patient in an altered state of consciousness often induced by hypnosis. Because of this altered state of consciousness and the material involved, this work can be classified as a type of transpersonal therapy, since it is beyond the bounds of normal, personal, waking consciousness. Since hypnosis is the tool of choice in doing this work, it is essential that the therapist be appropriately trained not only in hypnosis, but also hypnotherapy generally.

Historical considerations

Throughout history and in many cultures, there are references to spirit possession of one type or another. There are also descriptions of the casting out or releasing of these spirits in various ways. In traditional cultures, medicine men or shamans have usually performed these types of rituals. Descriptions of these rituals can be found in the anthropological literature. The rituals include such things as verbal formulae, herbal preparations, ritual movements, christening, etc.

In the Christian tradition, the casting out of spirits is well documented in the New Testament. Jesus cast out unclean spirits and exhorted the Apostles and disciples to do the same. There are many accounts in the writings of the early church fathers of spirit possession, battling spirits in the solitude of the desert in spiritual warfare, and of casting out of unclean spirits. The Catholic Church has a long history of exorcism.This ritual is still practiced around the world today by priests who are trained in the rite of exorcism.

Many other Christian denominations also practice exorcism and the casting out of spirits. This is usually more prevalent in charismatic or pentecostal denominations and movements. This is usually done with prayer, exhortation, and the laying on of hands.

Historically, in the various instances cited above, the demons or unclean spirits are usually just cast out of the person into the world at large, the outer darkness, or wherever. What distinguishes Spirit Releasement Therapy from this historical tradition is that in SRT, the spirits or entities are released into the Light. The underlying belief is that all beings are created by the Light and at center still have the original spark of Light. By focusing on this inner light, the entity can be drawn to the greater Light and released into this Light. The belief is that these entities are thus set free to continue their own evolution, or in the case of dark spirits, are saved or redeemed. This helps not only the patient who is freed from the influence of the entity, but also the entity who is freed to continue on in a more appropriate role. Sending the entity or spirit to the Light also prevents the entity or spirit from staying on the Earth plane and re-attaching to another person.

The phases of Spirit Releasement Therapy

Dr. Baldwin describes six phases of Spirit Releasement Therapy in his Technique Manual.[2] Since for the purposes of this chapter, we are considering this as a therapeutic technique rather than a therapy within itself, it needs to be emphasized that this technique would be appropriately used in the process of ongoing psychotherapy by a qualified mental health professional who has had hands on training in the use of this technique. In light of this, several other phases of treatment will be described along with Dr. Baldwin's six phases.

The first phase of treatment is part of any good psychotherapy and consists of a comprehensive clinical interview with the patient who is presenting for treatment. If the patient is coming with a request for Spirit Releasement Therapy, this interview is still a prerequisite and in many cases even of more crucial importance since many patients who are attracted to this type of therapy are not appropriate for it. For instance, patients with severe mental disorders may present for this type of treatment for a variety of reasons, e.g., they are resistant to and/or disillusioned with mainstream treatment, which may or may not have been appropriate and are seeking an alternative explanation for their symptoms and relief from those symptoms. These patients need to be appropriately diagnosed and treated, not naively treated with Spirit Releasement Therapy. Patients who are appropriate for this type of treatment will be identified as the treatment process unfolds through correct differential diagnosis.

Thus, the second phase of treatment consists of the beginning of the process of differential diagnosis and ruling out more conventional explanations for the patient's symptoms. At this point, it will have already been determined during the comprehensive clinical interview that the patient is exhibiting some symptoms that would suggest the possibility of entity attachment. Symptoms can include hearing inner voices, impulses to act in uncharacteristic ways, the sudden onset of unusual behaviors, and other personality changes, along with others types of symptoms that Dr. Baldwin describes in his technique manual. Other severe mental disorders are ruled out at this time using the mental health professional's diagnostic tools. Thus, such diagnoses as psychotic disorders, organically based or substance induced disorders, posttraumatic stress disorders, severe personality disorders, etc., are ruled out during this phase of differential diagnosis. Once this has been done, and the mental health professional decides that further differential diagnosis needs to be done using hypnosis, the next phase of treatment begins.

Exploring the patient's beliefs about hypnosis and thoroughly explaining hypnosis and hypnotherapy as well as explaining the process of continuing differential diagnosis is the third phase of treatment. This obviously assumes that the therapist is well trained in hypnosis generally and is qualified and licensed to practice this type of advanced therapeutic intervention. Once the patient is comfortable with the idea of hypnosis, it is often beneficial to do practice sessions with the patient, both to have them feel more comfortable with hypnosis and also to gauge their hypnotic ability. At least a moderate level of trance seems necessary to do this work with most people. Also, the professional explains to the patient that during hypnosis, the process of differential diagnosis will continue to further determine the cause of the patient's symptoms. This phase of differential diagnosis is mainly concerned with whether the patient again may have another mental disorder, such as a dissociative disorder of some type, or whether there may indeed be entity attachment of some type. But before moving on to the fourth phase of the technique of Spirit Releasement Therapy, I would like to give an example of the importance of differential diagnosis, and especially the need for exhaustive questioning. Thus, I would like to share the following clinical anecdote from my early experience with this type of therapy so others may learn from my mistakes.

A woman in her thirties presented for therapy with symptoms of depression. After several weeks of therapy, I noticed that she looked quite distracted at times. When I questioned her about this, she stated that voices were arguing within. After determining that these voices did not appear to be internal dialogue or auditory hallucinations, I discussed using hypnosis with her to get more information about these voices. The next session we did hypnosis and I began talking with someone who called herself by another name, claimed to be of a different age, and denied being part of the patient. Further, this someone denied ever having lived before, having been born with her own human body, etc. She affirmed that she had joined this woman at a particular point in her life. Based on these questions and some others, I hypothesized that this someone appeared to be an attached entity rather than an ego state or an alternate personality.

At the end of this session and during the next session, I discussed what I had found with the patient, its implications, and her beliefs in this area. Since this patient was quite intelligent, open minded, and was somewhat sophisticated in the areas of philosophy and spirituality, she could readily accept the possibility of entity attachment. So during the following session,

I again hypnotized her and talked with the entity. The entity again affirmed that she was not part of the patient. We then discussed that her attachment to this person was inappropriate and that I wished to help her be released to the Light so that she could continue her own soul development. She agreed to this. I then performed the spirit releasement, but to my dismay, it didn't work! I apologized to the entity, told her that we would speak again, and after alerting the patient, discussed what had occurred with her. We agreed to explore this further in the next session.

After further hypnosis and more extensive questioning of the entity, I finally determined that this was an alternate personality in a patient with severe Dissociative Identity Disorder who did not have a host personality and that none of her personalities admitted to being part of the patient. Rather, they all experienced themselves as being separate persons, with separate souls, who were trapped in this physical body. To them, the person who presented for therapy was a fiction they maintained for the outside world. Hopefully, this illustrates the clinical wisdom of proceeding slowly, doing extensive questioning, taking into account the possibility of delusions or lying, and clearly establishing a correct diagnosis before initiating therapeutic intervention.

In progressing to the fourth phase of treatment, after the patient is prepared and in a comfortable level of trance, the process of discovering and identifying any attached entities or spirits is started. As the professional continues the process of differential diagnosis, the possibility of a dissociative disorder needs to be thoroughly explored as illustrated in the example above. Once this is done, and there is further evidence of entity attachment, the professional now needs to discuss this possibility with the patient. It needs to be noted that entity attachment can and often does occur along with other mental disorders. Actually, these can be a predisposing factor in the sense of weakened ego boundaries and low ego strength that can facilitate entity attachment. For example, attachment may be facilitated by borderline personality organization, dissociative disorders, substance abuse disorders, and other disorders. Some proponents of this type of therapy believe that entity attachment is very widespread, e.g., 90 percent plus of the population. Whether this is actually the case is somewhat suspect at this time and would need to be further investigated. Also, some believe that more often than not, there is more than one entity attached to a person and that group releasements are necessary. This also would need further investigation and corroboration. Whatever the case may be, when an entity or spirit is discovered by responding through the patient, the next phase of treatment begins.

Thus, the fifth phase of treatment consists of discussing with the patient what has been found during hypnosis and the process of differential diagnosis. At this time, a person's religious, spiritual, and metaphysical beliefs need to be investigated as part of the ongoing therapeutic process in order to ascertain whether and how to approach the topic of entity attachment or spirit possession. If the patient is amenable to further exploring whether entity attachment or spirit possession might be the cause of their symptoms, and the choice of terminology can be crucial, then the therapist can proceed to the next phase of treatment. As part of this discussion, the possibility of entity attachment or spirit possession is discussed as well as the technique of Spirit Releasement Therapy.

As with any therapeutic intervention, the patient's informed consent is necessary to proceed with treatment. With Spirit Releasement Therapy, this informed consent is even more crucial, since for most patients, the hypothesis of spirit possession is likely to be unorthodox and unsettling at least, and possibly disruptive of their worldview and quite terrifying at most.

Once the therapist has completed the process of differential diagnosis, has explained to the patient the probability of spirit possession, and the process of Spirit Releasement Therapy, the sixth phase of treatment begins. Dr. Baldwin calls this phase of treatment dialoging with the spirit. Since this has already likely been occurring during differential diagnosis, it may be helpful to conceptualize this phase of treatment as negotiating and/or doing therapy with the entity or spirit. What takes place in this phase on treatment depends on the type of entity that is discovered and diagnosed. For instance, with an earthbound human spirit, an investigation of when and why the entity attached is usually conducted. The entity is reasoned with and convinced that it is really in their own and the patient's best interest for the entity to leave, go to the Light and continue their own soul evolution. Some type of therapy with the entity may be necessary to facilitate this release. If the entity is a discarnate, nonhuman entity of some type, other releasement techniques are utilized. For example, with a dark or demonic entity, a good deal of firm reasoning is necessary. It is also necessary to avoid ego or power struggles. The entity needs to understand that much of what it believes is a lie and be convinced to discover the Light within. Many are afraid of the Light and the Powers of Light may need to be invoked to help with the dark spirit. Much of what occurs in these cases entails a belief in and an understanding of the spiritual dimensions of reality. Without these necessary tools a therapist can easily become overwhelmed, frightened, and lost in the therapeutic process and possibly harm the patient or themselves. At this time, I would like to share another clinical anecdote to illustrate this technique.

This patient was an ongoing therapy patient who was recovering from chemical dependency. During the course of therapy, she related that teenage boys were repeatedly calling the house asking for a teenage girl named Emily. She and her husband had no idea who this might be. We had already used hypnosis in therapy, discussed her spiritual beliefs, etc. Thus, we proceeded to discuss exploring if this Emily might be some part of her, e.g., possibly an ego state that was operational during alcoholic blackouts, or possibly an attached entity. The patient agreed and under hypnosis, I talked with Emily. Emily related that she had attached herself to the patient when the patient was ten years old and very depressed. Emily said she was previously alive in her own human body and at death had become earthbound.

She had attached to the patient because of emotional resonance with her sadness and depression. I determined that Emily was an attached entity and not an ego state, alternate personality, etc. Emily had been with the patient all of these years, and as hypothesized above, did come out during alcoholic blackouts and called teenage boys.

After talking with Emily, I discussed what I had found with the patient who had spontaneous amnesia for this part of the session. This was unusual since she had always remembered the content of previous hypnotic sessions. The patient agreed with using Spirit Releasement Therapy (and in this case it was appropriate and worked). Emily was released to the Light, and eventually the phone calls stopped, along with the spontaneous disappearance of several other specific behaviors which the patient admitted were out of character, e.g., having a particular type of ice cream which she didn't like in the refrigerator and having it being eaten without her or her husband's knowledge.

The seventh phase of treatment is the actual releasing of the spirit or entity into the Light. Dr. Baldwin details many different types of techniques in his manual for releasing different types of spirits. With an earthbound human spirit, after whatever issues are holding them here are resolved as described in the phase above, they are then directed to focus on the Light. They usually begin to naturally move toward the Light. Also, the literature describes that most of the time they are met by other welcoming spirits from the Other Side. These are often friends or relatives who have gone before them. The released entity is escorted into the Light to continue their own evolution.

Releasing demonic entities or spirits can be much more difficult. Dr. Baldwin presents a twelve step sequence for releasing dark spirits in this technique manual. This often entails calling upon Angels of Light and Rescue Spirits to help with the work. This part of spirit releasement can strain or surpass the credulity of many therapists if they do not have a belief in and experience with the Inner Planes and Higher Order Beings. The language used in Dr. Baldwin's technique manual is generically Christian, referring to the Archangel Michael, the Legions of Heaven, etc. These supernatural entities are called on to capture and restrain the spirit for questioning, and also to escort the unwilling spirits to the Light. Much of this is seen as necessary for the therapist to avoid a power struggle with the demonic spirits. This technique assumes that the therapist does not have the power to cast out demons, but calls upon the Powers of the Light to help accomplish this task.

The next phase of treatment is very important in terms of protecting the patient from further harm and attachment, at least at the time. This eighth phase of treatment consists of doing a guided visualization with the patient to seal their energy field and prevent further spirit attachment. This visualization is a White Light meditation which surrounds and fills the patient with Light. This can be described as being bathed in the White Light, breathing in the White Light, letting it fill in the spaces left by the departing spirits or entities. The patient is encouraged to continue practicing this exercise for several days or weeks as needed. This phase completes the Spirit Releasement proper.

At this point, treatment continues with ongoing therapy. For most patients this will entail some type of processing and integration of the experience. This phase of therapy may also include discussing the significance of spirit attachment, how it can happen, and ways to avoid a recurrence. This can include talking about some form of prayer, meditation, rituals, etc. There are often distinct perceptual, attitudinal, and behavioral changes following a spirit releasement, and these will need to be processed and integrated by the patient. Such an experience can also profoundly impact on the patient's belief system, religious or otherwise, and these issues can be discussed in continuing therapy.

Conclusion

Spirit Releasement Therapy is an advanced therapeutic technique utilized with patients who have been diagnosed with a spirit attachment. Hypnosis is usually necessary to have the patient enter an altered state of consciousness to do this work. Thus, this technique can be classified as a type of transpersonal hypnotherapy. This type of work is most appropriately done by a qualified mental health professional who is trained in psychotherapy, hypnosis and hypnotherapy, differential diagnosis, and in the use of this technique specifically. This therapist should also be knowledgeable in metaphysics and spirituality, as well as having a worldview and belief system which can make understandable this type of work. Finally, the therapist needs to have his or her own personal spirituality which will provide a basis for this work and protection from spirit attachment.

As a final note, there is also a technique for Remote Depossession. This is described in Dr. Baldwin's technique manual as well as in a book by this name by Dr. Irene Hickman.[6] This technique involves the use of another person with psychic abilities to facilitate the process with the therapist. This technique has the same requirements as those described above for Spirit Releasement Therapy, plus training in the technique of Remote Depossession, and the availability of a willing, psychic facilitator.

In closing, SRT is an important transpersonal, therapeutic technique which is likely to gain greater acceptance in the near future. There will be a need for qualified and trained practitioners as more complementary and alternative forms of healthcare become more widely known and needed. As healthcare continues its present shift from a materialistic, reductionist paradigm to a more wholistic, transpersonal and spiritual paradigm, techniques such as SRT will be in demand.

References

1. Albertson, Maurice, et al., Post-Traumatic Stress Disorders of Vietnam Veterans: a proposal for research and therapeutic healing utilizing depossession, *J. Regression Ther.*, 3(1), Fall, 1988, 56–62.
2. Baldwin, William, *Spirit Releasement Therapy: a technique manual,* 2nd ed., The Human Potential Foundation Press, Los Angeles, 1993.
3. Baldwin, William, Report of a Study: Diagnosis and Treatment of the Spirit Possession Syndrome, *J. Regression Ther.*, VI(1), December, 1992, 48–61.
4. Denning, Hazel M., Two Cases of Depossession to Dissolve Anger, *J. Regression Ther.*, IV(2), October, 1990, 16–20.
5. Fiore, Edith, Freeing Stalemates in Relationships by the Resolution of Entity Attachments, *J. Regression Ther.*, 3(1), Fall, 1988, 22–25.
6. Hickman, Irene, *Remote Depossession*, Hickman Systems, 1994.
7. Ireland-Frey, Louise, Releasement of a Non–Human Entity: case report, *J. Regression Ther.*, VIII(1), December, 1994, 72–82.
8. Lucas, Winifred B., Spontaneous Remissions, *J. Regression Ther.*, 2(2), Fall 1987, 109–114.
9. Motoyama, Hiroshi, A Case of Possession in a Past Life Resulting in Physical Problems, *J. Regression Ther.*, 2(2), Fall, 1987, 108–109.
10. Silver, Carl, The New Age, The Mythic, and Legitimization of Regression/Releasement Therapy, *J. Regression Ther.*, VII(1), December, 1993, 73–79.
11. Vanella, Kristie, Self-Releasement of an Adolescent, *J. Regression Ther.*, IV(1), Spring, 1989, 73–74.

For further study:

Dr. William Baldwin
Center for Human Relations
P.O. Box 4061
Enterprise, FL 32725
http://www.spiritreleasement.org
email: Doctorbill@aol.com

chapter twelve

Cross-cultural perspectives on transpersonal hypnosis

Stanley Krippner

Transpersonal psychologists define their field as the study of experiences in which one's sense of identity extends beyond the personal to encompass wider, broader, higher, and/or deeper aspects of humankind, life, and the cosmos. Many other psychologists would agree that these experiences are worthy of study, even though they have been ignored by most mainstream psychologists over the years, despite William James' interest in the varieties of religious experiences and related human capacities. However, the transpersonalists have built an entire school of psychology around these reports and their implications, using them as the building blocks for a model of the complete person and his or her social environment. Typically, they insist that "the transpersonal model ... is not necessarily expected to replace or challenge the validity of earlier ones but rather to set them within an expanded context of human nature."[40] For me, transpersonal psychology is most usefully thought of as the disciplined study of behaviors and experiences that appear to transcend those hypothetical constructs associated with individual identities and self-concepts, as well as their developmental antecedents, and the implications of these behaviors and experiences for education, training, and psychotherapy.

Consciousness can be defined as the pattern of perception, cognition, and affect characterizing an organism at a particular period of time. Alterations in consciousness have been of great interest to transpersonalists because encounters with the divine, contact with the spirit world, and insights into the wider, broader, higher, and/or deeper aspects of existence typically occur during shamanic drumming, group dancing, meditation, and various states brought about by such plants as peyote and mind-altering cacti and mushrooms. Western observers have been reminded of hypnosis by some of these states, especially those in which individuals have seemed highly suggestible and externally motivated.

The term *hypnosis* is often used to refer to a variety of structured, goal-oriented procedures in which it is claimed that the suggestibility and/or motivation of an individual or a group is enhanced by another person (or persons), by a mechanical device, by a conducive environment, or by oneself. These procedures attempt to blur, focus, and/or amplify attention and/or mentation (e.g., imagination, intention) leading to the accomplishment of specified behaviors or experiences.[23]

Considerable research data indicate that these behaviors and experiences reflect expectations and role enactments on the part of the hypnotized individuals or groups who attend (often with little awareness) to their own personal needs and to the interpersonal or situational cues that shape their responses.[3,33] Other research data emphasize the part that attention (whether it is diffuse, concentrated, or expansive) plays in hypnosis, enhancing the salience of the suggested task or experience. Both these bodies of hypnosis literature emphasize the interaction of several variables in hypnosis, and can be utilized to better understand those healing practices used by native practitioners that involve either overt or covert suggestive and/or motivational procedures.

Historical and cross-cultural issues

The historical roots of hypnosis reach back to tribal rituals and the practices of native shamans. Agogino[2] states, "The history of hypnotism may be as old as the practice of shamanism," and describes hypnotic-like procedures used in the court of the Pharaoh Khufu in 3766 B.C. Agogino adds that priests in the healing temples of Asclepius (commencing in the 4th century, B.C.) induced their clients into "temple sleep" by "hypnosis and auto-suggestion," while the ancient Druids chanted over their clients until the desired effect was obtained (p. 32). Vogel[39] points out that herbs were used to enhance verbal suggestion by native healers in pre-Columbian Central and South America.

Gergen observes that the words by which the world is discussed and understood are social artifacts, "products of historically situated interchanges among people."[13] Therefore, I use the description "hypnotic-like procedures" because native (i.e., indigenous or traditional) practitioners and their societies have constructed an assortment of terms to describe activities that resemble what Western practitioners refer to as hypnosis. The term *hypnosis* has a cultural and historical context dating back to Franz Anton Mesmer in the 18th century. To indiscriminately use this term to describe exorcisms, the laying on of hands, dream incubation, etc., does an injustice to the varieties of cultural experience and their historic roots. "Hypnosis," "the hypnotic trance," and "the hypnotic state" have been reified too often, distracting the serious investigator from the ingenious uses of human imagination and motivation reported from many cultures that are worthy of study in their own terms.

A survey of the social science literature as well as my own observations in several traditional societies indicate that there are frequent elements of native healing procedures that can be termed hypnotic-like. This is due, in part, to the fact that alterations in consciousness (i.e., observed or experienced changes in people's patterns of perception, cognition, and/or affect at a given point in time) are not only sanctioned but are also deliberately fostered by virtually all indigenous groups. For example, Bourguignon and Evascu[5] read ethnographic descriptions of 488 different societies, finding that 89 percent were characterized by socially approved altered states of consciousness.

The ubiquitous nature of hypnotic-like procedures in native healing[6] is also the result of the ways in which human capacities, such as the capability to strive toward a goal and the ability to imagine a suggested experience, can be channeled and shaped, albeit differentially, by social interactions.[27] Concepts of sickness and of healing can be socially constructed and modeled in a number of ways. The models found in traditional (i.e., native) cultures frequently identify such etiological factors in sickness as soul loss and spirit possession, intrusion, or invasion, all of which are diagnosed (at least in part) by observable changes in the victims' behavior as related to their mentation or mood.[11] Unlike infectious diseases and disabilities resulting from physical trauma, these conditions, including many of those with a physiological predisposition, are socially constructed, just as the changed states of consciousness identified by Bourguignon and Evascu are shaped by historical and social forces within a culture.

For example, there is no Western equivalent for *wagamama*, a Japanese emotional disorder characterized by childish behavior, emotional outbursts, apathy, and negativity. Nor is there a counterpart to *kami*, a condition common in some Japanese communities that is thought to be caused by spirit possession. *Susto* is a malaise commonly referred to in Peru and several other parts of Latin America and thought to be caused by a shock or fright, often connected with breaking a spiritual taboo. It can lead to dire consequences such as the loss, injury, or wounding of one's soul, but there is no equivalent concept in Western psychotherapy manuals.

Cross-cultural studies of native healing have only started to take seriously the importance of understanding indigenous models of sickness and treatment, perhaps because of the prevalence of behavioral, psychoanalytic, and medical models, none of which have been overly sympathetic to the explanations offered by traditional practitioners or to the proposition that Western knowledge is only one of several viable representations of nature.[13] Kleinman[19] comments:

> The habitual (and frequently unproductive) way researchers try to make sense of healing, especially indigenous healing, is by speculating about psychological and physiological mechanisms of therapeutic action, which then are applied to case material in truly Procrustean fashion that fits the particular

> instance to putative universal principles. The latter are
> primarily derived from the concepts of biomedicine
> and individual psychology ... By reducing healing to
> the language of biology, the human aspects (i.e., psy-
> chosocial and cultural significance) are removed, leav-
> ing behind something that can be expressed in
> biomedical terms, but that can hardly be called healing.
> Even reducing healing to the language of behavior ...
> leaves out the language of experience, which ... is a
> major aspect of healing.

The value of a cross-cultural approach is to extend the range of individual and social variation in the scientific search for an understanding of
human capacities.[28] Therefore, in this chapter I will concentrate on describing
the use of hypnotic-like procedures for transpersonal purposes (using the
definitions of hypnosis and transpersonal already stated). Most illnesses in
a society are socially constructed, at least in part, and alleged changes in
consciousness also reflect social construction. Because native models of healing generally assume that practitioners, to be effective, must shift their attention and awareness (e.g., journeying to the upper world, traveling to the
lower world, incorporating spirit guides, conversing with power animals,
retrieving lost souls), the hypnosis literature can be instructive.

Western hypnotic models are often assumed to represent universal processes; however, this assumption is only partially correct. In the meantime,
native healing procedures are worthy of appreciation from the perspective
of their own social framework and need not be Westernized with the hypnosis label.

Hypnotic-like procedures in shamanism

Winkelman[41] conducted an archival study of 47 traditional societies, identifying four groups of spiritual practitioners: shamans and shamanic healers, priests and priestesses, mediums and diviners, and malevolent practitioners. With the exception of priests and priestesses, these practitioners
purportedly cultivated the ability to regulate and/or shift their patterns of
perception, affect, and cognition for benevolent (e.g., healing, divining) or
malevolent (e.g., casting spells, hexing) purposes. In addition, priests and
priestesses presided over rituals and ceremonies that often had, as their
intent, eliciting changes in the behavior and experiences of their supplicants
for religious purposes.

Transpersonal, hypnotic-like procedures are often apparent in the healing practices of native shamans. Shamans can be defined as socially sanctioned practitioners who purport to voluntarily regulate their attention and
awareness so as to access information not ordinarily available, using it to
facilitate appropriate behavior and healthy development, as well as to alleviate stress and sickness, among members of their community and/or for

the community as a whole. Among the shaman's many roles, that of healer is the most common. The functions of shamans may differ in various locations, but most of them have been called upon to predict and prevent afflictions, or to diagnose and treat them when they occur. Many of these procedures are transpersonal because they involve family and community members as well as facilitating altered states of consciousness in which the shaman and/or the client's sense of identity extends beyond the personal to encompass other dimensions of human experience.

Shamanic healing procedures are highly scripted in a manner similar to the way that hypnotic procedures are carefully sequenced and structured. The expectations of the shaman's or hypnotist's client can enable them to decipher task demands, interpret relevant communications appropriately, and translate the practitioner's suggestions into personalized perceptions and images. Just as expectancy plays a major role in hypnotic responsiveness,[18] it facilitates the responsiveness of shamans' clients as well as expediting shamanic "journeying." Shamans themselves display what Kirsch,[18] in discussing the hypnosis literature, calls "learned skills;" their introduction to hypnotic-like experiences during their initiation and training generalizes to later sessions, and they can ultimately engage in "journeying" virtually at will. For this reason, it is debatable whether shamanic journeying is a dissociative phenomena; there is no shift of the shaman's personal identity, and the shaman appears to be in control of the journeying process and does not incorporate the entities encountered along the way.

Japanese shamans of the Tohoku region believe that they can contact the Buddhist goddess Kan'non who assists with their diagnosis, producing visual or auditory imagery that the shaman experiences and reports. This is an example of the "translation" that characterizes both hypnotic sessions and shamanic imagination. These shamanic translations have been studied by Achterberg[1] who considers dreams, visions, and similar processes a venerable source of vital information on human health and sickness. So ubiquitous is their process of gleaning pertinent information from fantasy-based symbols and metaphors that I[20] have suggested that shamans, as a group, might be considered "fantasy prone." Indeed, they frequently resemble the highly hypnotizable individuals who, on the basis of interviews and personality tests, have been designated "fantasy prone."[26] However, to engage in fantasy is simply to exercise one's imagination, and this can be done without transcending one's sense of identity. Thus, fantasy prone individuals do not have experiences that can be labelled transpersonal each time they utilize their imagination.

Furst[12] has described procedures by which North American Indians once sought (and still seek) alternative states of consciousness: "psychoactive plants, animal secretions, fasting, thirsting, self-mutilation, exposure to the elements, sweat lodges, sleeplessness, incessant dancing, bleeding, plunging into ice-cold pools, and different kinds of rhythmic activity, self-hypnosis, meditation, chanting, and drumming." Furst uses non-Indian concepts (e.g., self-hypnosis, trance, meditation) that may not be directly comparable to the original experiences. Nevertheless, he goes on to describe the freedom that was typically given by North American Indian shamans to their clients to use "ecstatic trance" in order to determine their own relationship with the unseen forces of the universe. The analogous hypnotic practices here would be the various non-directive, permissive procedures in which hypnotized clients utilize their own fantasy and imagery to work toward the desired goals.[24]

Jilek writes that the Nanaimo Indians of Vancouver Island "fall unconscious" in order to incorporate the tutelary spirits necessary for healing to occur.[15] Rogers claims that the Alaskan Eskimo shaman's use of rhythmic drumming and monophonic chanting induces self-hypnosis (apparently because of their goal-directed nature) as well as placing the client "in a hypnotic trance in which the suggestions of recovery and cure are given."[31] In discussing the Ammassalik Eskimos of Eastern Greenland, Kalweit observes that their "continuous rubbing of stones against each other may be seen as a simple way of inducing a trance … The monotony, loneliness, and repetitive rhythmic movement join with the desire to encounter a helping spirit. This combination is so powerful that it erases all mundane thoughts and distracting associations."[17] Again, the use of Western concepts may be flawed descriptors for what actually occurs in these instances of remarkable behavior.

Belo[4] claimed to have observed similarities between the behavior of Balinese healers and that of hypnotized subjects. Although there was no trained observer of hypnosis on Belo's field trips, a hypnotic practitioner observed several of her films and claimed to notice similarities between hypnotic trance and mediumistic trance. In these otherwise useful descriptions, we can observe the proclivity of Western observers to use such terms as *hypnosis* and *trance* in describing shamanic procedures rather than simply making comparisons or utilizing the tribe's own explanations.

Kirsch's[18] discussion of the role of expectancies in hypnosis and psychotherapy is relevant to each of these cases. Hypnosis, like many culturally-based rituals, serves to shape and bolster relevant expectancies that reorganize consciousness and produce behavioral changes relevant to the goals of hypnotic subjects and shamanic clients. For example, the ideomotor behavior that often characterizes hypnosis (e.g., arms becoming heavier or lighter, fingers moving to denote positive or negative responses) resembles the postures, gestures, collapsing motions, and rhythmic movements that occur during many native rituals. In both instances, the participants claim that the movements occur involuntarily. Kirsch suspects that expectancy plays a major role, but admits that these responses are experienced as occurring automatically, without volition.

The absence of a formal "induction" does not prevent the client from becoming receptive to a suggestion and motivated to follow it, just as most, if not all, hypnotic phenomena can be evoked without hypnotic induction.[18] Contributing to this procedure is the multi-modal approach that characterizes Navajo chants, as well as their repetitive nature and the mythic content of the words which are easily deciphered by those clients well-versed in tribal mythology. Sandner describes how the visual images of the sand paintings and the body paintings, the audible recitation of prayers and songs, the touch of the prayer stick and the hands of the medicine man, the taste of the ceremonial musk and herbal medicines, and the smell of the chant incense "all combine to convey the power of the chant to the patient."[32] A *hataalii* (i.e., Navajo shaman) usually displays a highly developed dramatic sense in carrying out the chant but generally avoids the clever sleight of hand effects used by many other cultural healing practitioners to demonstrate their abilities to the community.

The Navajo chants are considered by Sandner[32] to facilitate suggestibility and shifts in attention through repetitive singing and the use of culture-specific mythic themes. These activities prepare participants and their community for healing sessions that may involve symbols and metaphors acted out by performers, enacted in purification rites, or executed in sand paintings composed of sand, corn meal, charcoal, and flowers, but destroyed once the healing session is over. Some paintings, such as those used in the Blessing Way chant are crafted from ingredients that have not touched the ground, e.g., flower petals. Once again, the client translates the symbols and metaphors, but usually without full awareness of the ongoing process.

Hypnotic-like procedures affect the mentation of both the *hataalii* and the client during the chant. Sandner[32] points out that the *hataalii's* performance empowers the client by creating a "mythic reality" through the use of chants, dances, and songs (often accompanied by drums and rattles), masked dancers, purifications (e.g., sweats, emetics, herbal infusions, ritual bathings, sexual abstinence), and sand paintings. Joseph Campbell described the colors of the typical sand painting as those "associated with each of the four directions" and a dark center, "the abysmal dark out of which all things come and back to which they go."[7] When appearances emerge in the painting, "they break into pairs of opposites."

In addition to the chants, there are other hypnotic-like, transpersonal healing procedures used by the Navajo *hataalii*, one of which is a prayer session. For example, sacred corn pollen may be sacrificed during a time of prayer in an attempt to foster the influence of the spirits needed to heal the client; this ritual must be performed perfectly and behind locked doors, often at the home of the client. The door to the darkened hogan is fastened "to prevent the prayer from escaping." Sharpened flints are used to expel the evil from both the client and the hogan. Topper[37] holds that these procedures reduce the client's symptoms at the same time as they stabilize the social and emotional condition of the community.

Topper's study of Navajo *hataalii* indicate that they raise their clients' expectations through the example they set of stability and competence. Politically, they are authoritative and powerful; this embellishes their symbolic value as transference figures in the psychoanalytic sense, representing "a nearly omniscient and omnipotent nurturative grandparental object."[37] Frank and Frank put it more directly; "The personal qualities that predispose patients

to a favorable therapeutic response are similar to those that heighten susceptibility to methods of healing in nonindustrialized societies, religious revivals,
experimental manipulations of attitudes, and administration of a placebo."[11]

When treating Navajo clients, suggestion and expectancy are bolstered
through reinforcing the client's belief in the power of the chant and its
symbols, a tight structuring of the ceremonial performance, repetition (especially in chants, songs, and prayers), physical exhaustion of the client, dra-
matization of a significant event in Navajo mythology, and on rare occasions
the use of mind-altering herbal substances (e.g., datura) to evoke a physical
effect that convinces the client that power is at work. The hypnotic-like
procedures strengthen the support by family and community members as
well as the client's identification with figures and activities in Navajo cultural
myths, both of which are powerful elements in the attempted healing. Most
of these procedures are spiritual, but are they transpersonal? Sandner[32] found
that his informants were insulted when it was suggested that Navajo *hataali*
change their state of consciousness to such an extent that their sense of
identity is lost; such a shift would distract the practitioners from the attention
to detail and the precise memory needed for a successful performance.

Hypnotic-like procedures in Bali

In contrast, on the island of Bali, Indonesia, there are many rituals and
ceremonies that are transpersonal in nature and that utilize hypnotic-like
procedures. In traditional Balinese practice, the name of the main temple
ceremony is *nyimpen* and the dance of Calon Arang often is performed during
nyimpen. The story of Calon Arang revolves around an evil widow and her
only daughter who were banned to the forest for allegedly practicing black
magic. There are several variations of this story but all center around her
revenge against the people of the ancient Hindu Javanese kingdom of Daha
after its Raja insults her by retracting an offer to marry her beautiful daughter.
Calling up her demon legions, she transforms herself into a frightening figure
with ponderous hanging breasts, bulging eyes, a long flamed tongue, and a
mass of unruly flowing hair. Waving her magic cloth, she has become
Rangda, the queen of the witches, and wreaks havoc with her powers.
Understandably, this is one of the most powerful plays in sacred Balinese
drama and its performance is always charged with energy.

When I saw this dance performed, the dancers seemed oblivious to the
outside world and they enacted the great battle between the forces of the witch
and those of humankind. It started with the lesser characters whom, when
faced with defeat, called upon the aid of higher forces which transformed
them into more powerful beings. Each of the succeeding transformations was
met with mounting tension on the faces of the crowd. Children who were
dozing suddenly woke up. The climax finally came when the Barong, a mythical creature who frequently comes to the aid of human beings, at last faces
his arch-adversary, the malevolent witch Rangda, and the dancers shift from
their usual sense of identity to become players in this cosmic drama.

Thong,[36] a psychiatrist who organized the first mental hospital on Bali, describes what occurred during a performance of this dance that he witnessed:

> At that very moment, one of my staff was bringing to me another glass of the thick Balinese coffee that I had been using to keep from falling in sleep at that late hour. Suddenly, without warning, he threw the glass over his shoulder, stood upright as if in anger, and quivered with wide open eyes. Abruptly he proceeded to turn and walk to a nearby papaya tree which he pulled out of the ground. That seems to have been some sort of signal because afterwards many others in the crowd, including a member of the orchestra, experienced the same radical transformation. My first frightening impression was that utter chaos had broken out.

Overwhelmed by this sudden and unexpected turn of events, Thong sat confused and bewildered with no idea of where to look or what to do. Fortunately, the Balinese themselves had no such problem. Restraining the disorderly behavior of the more violent of the entranced dancers, their attention focused once more on the stage and its surroundings. The players still were dancing, still in an altered state of consciousness, but one that was less intense. Thong's most striking observation was that despite all the wailing and untamed antics, nobody was hurt.

> This led me to the conclusion that this was no true chaos; instead it was a wild but nonetheless orderly form of behavior. It was only at this point that I turned around to ask my Western companion, Christopher, a question about his feelings concerning this primal scene. The result was my second shock of the night when I saw Christopher sitting upright with the same dazed look in his eyes as the dancers. At that moment...all the trancers gathered before the Barong who began to lead a procession around the temple. Dear Christopher joined in as well.

It took the efforts of a *pemangku*, or village priest, to gently bring Christopher and the other people back to their ordinary state of consciousness. With his assistants, and armed only with holy water, the *pemangku* wandered through the crowd sprinkling the entranced revelers; the sacred water quickly revived them. Could this phenomenon be categorized as mass hypnosis? Such a label would be less than accurate because there was no formal hypnotic induction or direct goal-orientation of the entranced individuals.

Some of the most dramatic transformations of consciousness among children I have seen were in Bali. One evening, I watched the *Sanghyang Dedari*, a form of *Legong*, the "dance of revered angels," performed by two young girls after they supposedly had incorporated benevolent spirits. Enveloped by the smell of sweet incense and accompanied by the music of both an all-male chorus and an all-female chorus chanting sacred songs, the two girls moved rhythmically with their eyes closed, thus protecting their beloved temple from malevolent entities. The girls danced in flawless tandem, never opening their eyes but, perhaps, carefully responding to the music, to kinesthetic cues, and to memory. Once the chanting ended, the girls fell to the ground and were attended to by the *pemangku*, the village priest.

I have also seen the *Sanghyang Jaran*, during which boys and adolescents enter altered states and dance on a bamboo hobbyhorse or simply on a tree branch. Initially, they dance around a bonfire made from coconut husks, but if the spirit so dictates, they dance through the fire, often stepping on the burning husks and the coals. It is claimed that neither type of dancer has had any formal dance training; the participants insist that they cannot recall the dance steps once the priest brings them out of their altered state.

Another traditional performance, the Balinese *Kecak* dance, tells a story from the Hindu Ramayana collection. Sita is captured by the abhorrent Rawana but is rescued by Hanuman and his indomitable monkey army. At one point a circle of some 150 men provide incredibly coordinated movements, and their vocalizations, *Chak-Chak-Chak*, are remarkable imitations of monkey chatter. The purpose of the *Kecak* dance is to drive away Rawana and his evil spirits; in so doing, individual awareness gives way to a transpersonal group awareness.

In Thong's[36] opinion, the Balinese people's repressed emotions find an outlet in the dance and drama, an outlet the culture has provided for them to abreact, either vicariously or directly. Classical dance and drama in Bali, based on legends and myths, are well attended and the more contemporary dramatic presentations are even more widely attended. In both the classical and contemporary performing arts one can encounter every possible Balinese emotion, e.g., love, joy, anger, reverence. One can observe intrigue, sexual passion, jealousy, and the violation of all the cultural taboos. Not only do the players benefit from expressing these emotions and breaking the taboos, but the audience attains catharsis as well. From Thong's perspective, the other Balinese arts — painting, sculpture, the creation of festival offerings — help the Balinese to maintain a healthy frame of mind. They have retained their vitality; without them and the related cultural manifestations, the uniqueness of Bali would have crumbled long ago.

In addition, I have seen *balians* (i.e., Balinese shamans) enter both transpersonal and non-transpersonal altered states during healing and exorcism ceremonies. The *balian taksu* is a healer with mediumship talent who alters consciousness to assist in the diagnosis of the ill and unfortunate. Sometimes, the diagnosis is *bebai* in which an evil spirit has been sent by a sorcerer. The victim's rival has paid the sorcerer to practice *bebainan*, or black magic, for purposes of revenge or jealousy.[4] Thong concluded that in the "altruistic trance states," a dancer responds to the needs of another person or a group of people. This state is usually reached during or after the performance of a ritual and, in Bali, would encompass all hypnotic-like phenomena during religious or healing ceremonies as practiced by the *balian*. The practitioners in this group rarely show signs of psychopathology. Egoistic trance states, on the other hand, are entered in response to an individual's personal needs. They are not preceded by a ritual and tend to occur spontaneously. In Bali, this state is believed to be brought about by the possession of an individual by a *bebai* or evil spirit. Members of this group usually have emotional problems that typically fall into the psychiatric category of hysterical reaction. In other words, Thong's altruistic trance state is likely to be transpersonal in nature while the egoistic trance state is not.

Taking a transpersonal approach, Thong concluded that in Balinese ritualistic dancing, the "I" gives way to a loss of ego boundaries and a change in the body image. It was his hunch that some of the dances, such as the dreamy *sanghyang*, are states of hypoarousal, while others, such as the *Barong*, are states of hyperarousal. Indeed, the *Barong* dance, in both its original and tourist version, ends with the dancers pressing kris knives against their chests as the malevolent Rangda attempts to influence the dancers to harm themselves. The *Barong*, however, offers them protection. Thong determined that these hypnotic-like experiences could be divided into three stages. During the first stage, dancers are consciously or unconsciously preparing themselves; they have not yet lost reflective consciousness and still retain voluntary control and decision-making capabilities. The second stage brings intensification at which time control is lost and consciousness is altered. During the third stage, the dancer falls into a stage of exhaustion but may be capable of returning to the second stage if sufficiently aroused. The change from one stage to another can usually be recognized by distinct somatic clues such as sighs, sobs, hisses, shouts, or body movements.

Incense and scents are a common means of altering consciousness, but they seem to be incidental in Bali. Mind-altering substances such as psychedelic plants, alcohol, and even betel nut and tobacco play little or no role in Bali, despite the presence of psychedelic mushrooms (*jamur tahi sapi* in Balinese) on the island. The effects of the mushrooms are referred to as *lengehin* or dizziness; they are shunned by most Balinese who have a cultural dislike of anything that disorients them and threatens their sense of balance. In Thong's opinion, the most important factor is the charged and expectant atmosphere that surrounds altering consciousness. In other words, the social setting and expectancy seem to be more critical than any physiological maneuver. The leaders of the community play an important role because it is often the head of the village, the *sadeg*, or some other important personage who first goes into an altered state, serving as a role model for the others.

Perhaps the occurrence of hypnotic-like procedures cross-culturally is so frequent because it plays an important cultural role. In Bali, trance dancing serves as a useful emotional outlet both for the dancer and the observer.

What Thong calls altruistic trance states are preceeded by a ritual or ceremony in which a transpersonal shift is expected and accepted as an integral element. The trancers in these dances are usually ordinary members of the community with no more than the average number of psychological or physical problems. These ceremonies facilitate social cohesion because they are performed on behalf of the entire community.

What Thong calls egoistic trance states occur outside the ordinary cultural context. They may involve malicious magical practices, in which attempts are made (or are perceived to have been made) to influence, coerce, or harm community members. These trancers show a tendency for attacks of hysteria, acute psychotic reactions, and schizophrenic episodes. The Balinese themselves recognize these two types of trancers and react differently toward each of them.

Afro-Brazilian healing procedures

Transpersonal experiences were common in early West African cultures where individuals were considered to be closely connected with nature, the community, and their communal group. Each person was expected to play his or her part in a web of kinship relations and community networks. Strained or broken social relations were held to be the major cause of sickness; a harmonious relationship with one's community, as well as with one's ancestors, was important for health. At the same time, an ordered relationship with the forces of nature, as personified by the *orixas*, or deities, was essential for maintaining the well-being of the individual, the family, and the community. West Africans knew that disease often had natural causes, but believed that these factors were exacerbated by discordant relationships between people and their social and natural milieu. Long before Western medicine recognized the fact, Africa's traditional healers took the position that ecology and interpersonal relations affected people's health.[29]

West African healing practitioners felt that they gained access to supernatural power in three ways: by making offerings to the *orixa*, by foretelling the future with the help of an *orixa*, and by incorporating an *orixa* (or even an ancestor) who then diagnosed illnesses, prescribed cures, and provided the community with warnings or blessings. The medium, or person through whom the spirits spoke and moved, performed this task voluntarily, claiming that such procedures as dancing, singing, or drumming were needed to surrender their minds and bodies to the discarnate entities.[21] The slaves brought these practices to Brazil with them; despite colonial and ecclesiastical repression, the customs survived over the centuries and eventually formed the basis for a number of robust Afro-Brazilian spiritual movements. Books by a French spiritist, Alan Kardec, were brought to Brazil, translated into Portuguese, and became the basis for a related movement (i.e., Kardecism). There were followers of Mesmer in this group, but Kardec proposed that spirits, rather than Mesmer's invisible fluids, were the active agent in altering consciousness, removing symptoms, and restoring equilibrium.[30]

Contemporary *iyalorixas*, or "mães dos santos" (mothers of the saints), and *babalawos*, or "pais dos santos" (fathers of the saints), still teach apprentices how to sing, drum, and dance in order to incorporate the various deities, ancestors, and spirit guides. They also teach the *iãos* (children of the *orixas*) about the special herbs, teas, and lotions needed to restore health, and about the charms and rituals needed to prevent illness. The ceremonies of the various Afro-Brazilian groups (e.g., Candomblé, Umbanda, Batuque, Caboclo, Quimbanda, Xango) differ, but all share three beliefs: humans have a spiritual body (that generally reincarnates after physical death); discarnate spirits are in constant contact with the physical world; humans can learn how to incorporate spirits for the purpose of healing.

After interviewing 40 spiritistic healing practitioners in Brazil, I identified five methods of receiving the "call" to become a medium:[21]

1. coming from a family having a history of mediumship
2. being "called" by spirits in one's visions and dreams
3. succumbing to a malady or spiritual crisis from which one recovers in order to serve others
4. having a revelation while reading Afro-Brazilian spiritistic literature or attending spiritistic worship services
5. working as a volunteer in a spiritistic healing center and becoming inspired by the daily examples of compassion.

If the call is rejected, severe illness or misfortune may result; as one Candomble medium told me, "Once the *orixa* calls, there is no other path to take." In this case, the transpersonal dimension of human existence is recognized as so sacred and inviolate that one dare not reject its summons.

Once the apprentices begin to receive instruction in mediumship, such experiences as spirit incorporation, automatic writing, out-of-body travel, and recall of past lives lose their bizarre quality and seem to occur quite naturally. Socialization processes provide role models and the support of peers. A number of cues (songs, chants, music, etc.) facilitate spirit incorporation, and a process of social construction teaches control, appropriate role-taking, and communal support. Richeport[30] observed several similarities between these mediumistic behaviors and those of hypnotized subjects, e.g., suggestibility, the positive use of imagination, occasional amnesia for the experience.

It should be noted that mediums resemble shamans in many ways but lack the control of their attention and awareness that characterizes shamans. For example, shamans are usually aware of everything that occurs while they converse with the spirits, even when a spirit "speaks through" them. Mediums claim to lose awareness once they incorporate a spirit, and purport to remember little about the experience once the spirit leaves. Both shamans and mediums engage in altered states of consciousness, but the shaman's attention, memory, and awareness seem to be enhanced, not restricted. These same facets of mentation appear to be dampened or diffused in mediumship; if there is a shift toward greater focus, it is attributed to the guiding spirit rather than to the medium himself or herself, hence lending itself to the transpersonal description.

The traits most admired in mediums resemble those traits that facilitate ordinary social interactions. During more than a dozen exploratory trips to Brazilian healing centers, I have observed few instances of bizarre behavior during spiritistic ceremonies. Indeed, if a spirit seems to be taking control of the medium too quickly, the other mediums may sing a song that will slow down the process of incorporation. Leacock and Leacock[25] observed that the Brazilian mediums in their study usually behaved in ways that were "basically rational," communicated effectively with other people, and demonstrated few symptoms of hysteria or psychosis. They engaged in intensive training and, as mediums, pursued hard work that often put them at risk with seriously ill individuals. These are not likely to be the favorite pastimes of fragile personalities or malingerers.

In 1973, a colleague and I attended an Umbanda ceremony in Sao Paulo, Brazil. Drums were beating, candles were flickering, and the smell of incense was wafting through the room. We took our seats with the other spectators, and noticed the gargantuan altar containing dozens of statues of *orixas*, ancestors, and Christian saints — Umbanda being the Afro-American spiritistic movement that has borrowed most heavily from Christianity. A *babalawo* appeared to be in charge of the ceremony, but four other *babalawos* and five *orixas* were playing prominent roles.

As the ceremony continued, a medium began to shake violently, then appeared to demonstrate equanimity as she incorporated the spirit of a *preto velho*, a black slave from Brazil's colonial past. Looked upon as powerful healing spirits, the *preto velhos* are incorporated at least once a month in most Afro-Brazilian spiritistic centers, rotating with such other healing entities as the *caboclos*, or Indians of mixed blood, and the *crianças*, or children who died at young ages.

Other mediums began to engage in automatisms, twitching, writhing, screaming, flailing, and falling to the floor. Once they maintained their composure, they claimed to have incorporated *preto velhos*, and were able to engage in healing through the laying on of hands. My colleague and I entered the healing circle where mediums prayed, sang, and gave us brief massages that were pleasant and pleasurable. (Some spiritistic healers, especially the followers of Alan Kardec, only work with the spiritual body and refrain from touching the client's physical body.) It was not long before many recipients of the healing procedures began to display hypnotic-like behaviors including automatisms, conversations with the spirits, and spontaneous chanting and singing.

As the ceremony ended, obeisance was paid to the *exus*, or messengers of the *orixas*; these entities can be mischievous and so must be placated before the session, after the session, or both if the maximum results are to be obtained. Songs, prayers, and offerings of food and drink are sent their way to cajole them and insure their cooperation. Soon the mediums left the room, doffed their white robes and crucifixes, and joined us for refreshments. They alleged not to have recalled the events of the evening, claiming that as the *pretos velhos* had started to work through them, they lost their awareness of the ongoing activities.

In 1991, with several colleagues, I attended a *Candomblé* ceremony in the Centro Espirita of Recife, finding ourselves immersed in candlelight, incense, and drumming. *Pai Ely,* the founder of the Center and a "father of the saints," had invited us to witness an initiation: a "daughter of the temple" was about to become an *ião,* a *filha-de-santo* or "daughter of the saints." This followed a three-week period of solitude in an isolated room (the *ronco*) where her only visitor had been *Pai Ely* who had brought food, water, and counsel. As she emerged from the *ronco,* we noticed that her head had been shaved (the *raspagem da cabeça),* except for a thin tuft of hair in the middle of her head. We were told that this represented a modification of the original ceremony where the skin on top of the head was cut so that the *orixas* could receive a blood offering.

For several hours, we observed the initiate dance around the central open space of the Centro Espirita, accompanied by other mediums who were letting various entities "inhabit" their bodies. Some of them had been initiated years earlier, and continued to venerate the *orixas* who guided the initiates. For some it was Oxum, the *orixa* of the fresh water lakes and rivers; for others, it was Oxossi, the *orixa* of the forests. Having been silent for so long, the initiate's first words would be her *proclamação de nome,* the proclamation that would confirm the *orixa* who had served as her benefactor. Later that evening, the young woman gave us the name, "Oxumaré," the "rainbow *orixa*"who presides over life's transitions. The initiate was then welcomed as the temple's newest "daughter of the saints."

Later I discovered that Oxumaré is a man for six months, a woman for six months, and links the earth to the sky. We were told that what we had witnessed was a *saida de ião* ceremony in which the "daughter of the temple" finally "comes out" of her seclusion. It cumulates when the *orixa* whispers a special name (i.e., *dar o nome).* It was my understanding that the *ião* we observed already knew that she was a member of the Oxumaré lineage. However, there are many Oxumarés; old ones, young ones, female versions, male versions, Northern Brazil Oxumarés, Southern Brazil Oxumarés; in other words, Oxumarés come in all the colors of the rainbow. The particular identity of this initiate's Oxumaré was a vital part of this ceremony and of the social construction of the new *ião.* Further, the entire process exemplifies three phrases quite common to initiation ceremonies, namely separation (the initiate's selection), immersion (her three-week period of solitude), and return (her public dance and the giving of her name).

In both of these ceremonies, and in dozens of others that I have witnessed or in which I have participated, a trance was supposedly induced by the rhythmic drumming and movement as well as by the assault on the senses produced by the music, incense, flickering candles, and in some temples, pungent cigar smoke. But it was apparent to me that powerful demand characteristics were also at work. The very reason for the mediums' presence was the incorporation of spirits; as Kleinman argues, "providing effective treatment for disease is *not* the chief reason why indigenous practitioners heal. To the extent that they provide culturally legitimated treatment of illness, they *must* heal."[19]

In addition, the community of believers depended on the mothers, fathers, and children of the *orixas* to provide a connection to the spirit world that would ensure the well-being of the temple, prevent illness among those who were well, and bestow healing upon those who were indisposed. When one medium incorporated an *orixa*, *preto velho*, *caboclo*, or *criança*, an entire series of incorporations soon followed, domino-like. Just as many participants in hypnotic sessions seem eager to present themselves as "good subjects,"[33] the mediums in Afro-Brazilian healing sessions may be eager to present themselves as "good mediums," and to enact behaviors consistent with this interpretation. I have also noticed that the presence of visitors appears to increase both the speed and the dramatic qualities of spirit incorporation.

A fairly consistent similarity among mediums is their supposed inability to recall the events of the incorporation after the spirits have departed. However, Spanos has pointed out that this amnesic quality could just as easily be explained as an "achievement;" each failure to remember "adds legitimacy to a subject's self-presentation as 'truly unable to remember'," hence as deeply in "trance."[33] In other words, the interpretation of hypnotic phenomena as goal-directed action is helpful in understanding mediumship as an activity that meets role demands, as mediums guide and report their behavior and experience in conformance with these demands. It may not be that they lose control over the behavior as they incorporate a spirit, but rather that they engage in a efficacious enactment of a role that they are eager to maintain.

An alternative point of view would hold that the mediums actually do lose control over their behavior, entering a trance or dissociative state that allows hidden parts of themselves to manifest as secondary personalities or, in the case of the Brazilian mediums, as spirits. But some Brazilian practitioners with whom I have discussed these issues suggest that both the role-playing and dissociative paradigms merely describe the mechanism by which a medium actually incorporates the *orixa*, discarnate entity, or spirit. It is the incorporation itself, and the subsequent behavior of the spirit, that represent the crux of mediumship. Because the possibility of spirit incorporation can hardly be demonstrated at the present time, one can simply acknowledge this argument (albeit skeptically) and focus on other aspects of these phenomena.

For example, Afro-Brazilian spiritistic ceremonies enable clients and mediums to arrive at a shared world view in which an ailment can be discussed and treated.[38] In some spiritistic traditions, there are mediums who specialize in diagnosis, mediums who specialize in healing by a laying on of hands, mediums who specialize in distant healing, and mediums who specialize in intercessory prayer. Treatment may also consist of removing a "low spirit" from a client's "energy field," integrating one's past lives with the present incarnation, the assignment of prayers or service-oriented projects, or referral to a homeopathic physician. All of these procedures contain the possibility of enhancing clients' sense of mastery, increasing their self-healing capacities, and replacing their demoralization with empowerment.[11,38]

The mediums are not the only ones who appear to manifest hypnotic-like effects. Their clients also demonstrate apparent shifts in consciousness, especially while undergoing crude surgeries without the benefit of anes-thetics; however, Greenfield[14] has observed that the Brazilian mediums make no direct effort to alter their clients' awareness. Greenfield, who attributes the benefits of these sessions to the clients' alterations of con-sciousness, has observed that "no one is consciously aware of hypnotizing ... patients, ... and unlike the mediums, patients participate in no ritual during which they may be seen to enter a trance state." However, there are a number of cultural procedures that Greenfield found to be hypnotic-like in nature. One of them is the relationship of client and healer, characterized by trust, and resembling "that between hypnotist and client" in that these clients act positively in response to what the medium tells them. Another procedure is the provision of a context that allows the client to become totally absorbed in the intervention, a healing ritual that galvanizes the client's attention and distracts him or her from feeling pain. Greenfield adds that the spiritistic aspects of Brazilian culture foster "fantasy proneness" because large numbers of people believe that supernatural entities are help-ing (or hindering) them in their daily lives.

Rogers[31] has divided native healing procedures into several categories:

- nullification of sorcery (e.g., charms, dances, songs)
- removal of objects (e.g., sucking, brushing, shamanic "surgery")
- exorcism of harmful entities (e.g., fighting the entity, sending a spirit to fight the entity, making the entity uncomfortable)
- retrieval of lost souls (e.g., by "soul catchers," by shamanic journeying)
- eliciting confession and penance (e.g., to the shaman, to the community)
- transfer of illness (e.g., to an object, to a "scapegoat")
- suggestion and persuasion (e.g., reasoning, use of ritual, use of herbs)
- shock (e.g., sudden change of temperature, precipitous physical assault)

There are hypnotic-like segments of these procedures that utilize symbols, metaphors, stories, and rituals, especially those involving group participation.

Discussion

Hypnosis is a noun while *hypnotic-like* and *transpersonal* are adjectives, hence the use of the former term lends itself to abuse more easily than utilization of the latter terms. This distinction is important when one reads such accounts as that by Torrey who surveyed indigenous psychotherapists, concluding, on the basis of anecdotal reports, that "many of them are effective psychotherapists and produce therapeutic change in their clients."[38] Torrey observed that when the effectiveness of psychotherapy paraprofessionals has been studied, professionals have not been found to demonstrate superior therapeutic skills. The sources of that effectiveness are the four basic components of psychotherapy: a shared world view, personal qualities of the healer, client expectations, and a process that enhances the client's learning and mastery. I would suggest that an adjective such as "psychotherapist-like" would be a more accurate term that Torrey's use of the noun "psychotherapist" in describing native practitioners. I am more comfortable with Strupp's description as it uses nouns consistently: "The modern psychotherapist ... relies to a large extent on the same psychological mechanisms used by the faith healer, shaman, physician, priest, and others, and the results, as reflected by the evidence of therapeutic outcomes, appear to be substantially similar."[34]

Especially valuable are qualitative analyses of the experiences of both practitioners and their clients. I have used questionnaires[22] to study perceived long-term effects following visits to Filipino and Brazilian folk healers, finding such variables as "willingness to change one's behavior" to significantly correlate with reported beneficial modifications in health. Cooperstein interviewed 10 prominent alternative healers in the United States, finding that their procedures involved the self-regulation of their "attention, physiology, and cognition, thus inducing altered awareness and reorganizing the healer's construction of cultural and personal realities."[8] Cooperstein concluded that the concept that most closely represented his data was "the shamanic capacity to transcend the personal self, to enter into multiform identifications, to access and synthesize alternative perspectives and realities, and to find solutions and acquire extraordinary abilities used to aid the community." Indeed, the shaman's role and that of the alternative healer are both socially constructed, as are their operating procedures and their patients' predispositions to respond to the treatment. It is not only important to study the effects of the hypnotic-like procedures found in native healing, but to accurately describe them, and understand them within their own framework.

The professionalization of shamanic and other traditional healers demonstrates their similarity to practitioners of Western medicine.[10] Nevertheless, the differences cannot be ignored. Rogers has contrasted the Western and native models of healing, noting that in Western medicine, "Healing procedures are usually private, often secretive. Social reinforcement is rare... The cause and treatment of illness are usually regarded as secular... Treatment may extend over a period of months or years."[31] In native healing, however, "Healing procedures are often public: many relatives and friends may attend the rite. Social reinforcement is normally an important element. The shaman speaks for the spirits or the spirits speak through him [or her]. Symbolism and symbolic manipulation are vital elements.

Healing is of limited duration, often lasting but a few hours, rarely more than a few days."

Rogers has also presented three basic principles that underlie the native approach to healing: The essence of power is such that it can be controlled through incantations, formulas, and rituals; the universe is controlled by a mysterious power that can be directed through the meticulous avoidance of certain acts and through the zealous observance of strict obligations toward persons, places, and objects; the affairs of humankind are influenced by spirits, ghosts, and other entities whose actions, nonetheless, can be influenced to some degree by human effort.[31] This worldview, which fosters the efficacy of hypnotic-like procedures, varies from locale to locale but is remarkably consistent across indigenous cultures. The ceremonial activities produce shifts of attending for both the healer and the client. The culture's rules and regulations produce a structure in which the clients' motivation can operate to empower them and stimulate their self-healing aptitudes.

Western practitioners of hypnosis utilize the same human capacities that have been used by native practitioners in their hypnotic-like procedures. These include the capacity for imaginative suggestibility, the ability to shift attentional style, the potential for intention and motivation, and the capability for self-healing made possible by neurotransmitters, internal repair systems, and other components of mind/body interaction. These capacities often are evoked in ways that resemble Ericksonian hypnosis[9] because of their emphasis on narrative accounts. Hypnosis and hypnotic-like activities are complex and interactive, and hence take different forms in different cultures. Yet, as with other forms of therapy, "the mask ... crafted by the group's culture will also fit a majority of its members."[16] Transpersonal considerations are more common in the non-Western cultures I have surveyed or visited; to refer to traditional rituals and ceremonies as hypnosis can lead to a devaluing of these transpersonal elements.

It has become increasing apparent to cross-cultural psychologists that the human psyche cannot be extricated from the historically variable and diverse "intentional worlds" in which it plays a co-constituting part. Supposedly, writing makes reality accessible by representing consensual reality, but far too often it becomes a substitute for the reality it purports to represent. Therefore, I am dismayed when I see Western terms haphazardly applied to indigenous practices; for example, *amok* in Indonesia has been called "a trance-like state" and *latah* "a condition akin to hysteria."[35] By investigating ways in which different societies have constructed diagnostic categories and remedial procedures, therapists and physicians can explore novel and vital changes in their own procedures, hypnotic and otherwise, that have become obdurate and rigid. Western medicine and psychotherapy have their roots in traditional practices and need to explore avenues of potential cooperation with native practitioners of healing methods that may still contain wise insights and practical applications.

References

1. Achterberg, J., *Imagery in healing: shamanism and modern medicine*, Shambhala, Boston, 1985.
2. Agogino, G.A., The use of hypnotism as an ethnologic research technique, *Plains Anthropologist*, 10, 31–36, 1965.
3. Barber, T.X., *Hypnosis: a scientific approach*, Van Nostrand Reinhold, New York, 1969.
4. Belo, J., *Trance in Bali*, Columbia University Press, New York, 1960.
5. Bourguignon, E., and Evascu, T., Altered states of consciousness within a general evolutionary perspective: a holocultural analysis, *Behavior Science Research*, 12, 199–216, 1977.
6. Bowers, M.K., Hypnotic aspects of Haitian voodoo, *Int. J. Clin. Exper. Hypnosis*, 9, 269–282, 1961.
7. Campbell, J., *Transformations of Myth Through Time*, Harper & Row, New York, 1990.
8. Cooperstein, M.A., The myths of healing: a summary of research into transpersonal healing experience, *J. Am. Soc. Psychical Res.*, 86, 99–133, 1992.
9. Erickson, M.H., Rossi, E.L., and Rossi, S.H., *Hypnotic realities: the induction of clinical hypnosis and the indirect forms of suggestion*, Irvington, New York, 1976.
10. Feinstein, D. and Krippner, S., *The Mythic Path*, Tarcher/Putnam, New York, 1997.
11. Frank, J.D. and Frank, J.B., *Persuasion and Healing*, 3rd ed., Johns Hopkins University Press, Baltimore, 1991.
12. Furst, P.T., "High states" in culture-historical perspective, in *Alternate states of consciousness*, N.E. Zinberg, Ed., 53–88, Free Press, New York, 1977.
13. Gergen, K.J., The social constructionist movement in modern psychology, *Am. Psychol.*, 40, 266–275, 1985.
14. Greenfield, S.M., Hypnosis and trance induction in the surgeries of Brazilian spiritist healer-mediums, *Anthropology of Consciousness*, 2(3–4), 20–25, 1992.
15. Jilek, W.G., *Indian Healing: shamanic ceremonialism in the Pacific Northwest today*, Hancock House, Blaine, WA, 1982.
16. Kakar, S., *Shamans, Mystics and Doctors: a psychological inquiry into India and its healing traditions*, Knopf, New York, 1982.
17. Kalweit, H., *Dreamtime and Inner Space: the world of the shaman*, Shambhala, Boston, 1988.
18. Kirsch, I., *Changing Expectations: a key to effective psychotherapy.*, Brooks/Cole, Pacific Grove, CA, 1990.
19. Kleinman, A., *Patients and healers in the context of culture*, University of California Press, Berkeley, 1980.
20. Krippner, S., Dreams and shamanism, in *Shamanism: An expanded view of reality*, S. Nicholson, Ed., 125–132), Wheaton, IL, Theosophical Publishing, 1987.
21. Krippner, S., A call to heal: patterns of entry in Brazilian mediumship, in *Altered states of consciousness and mental health: a cross-cultural perspective*, C. Ward, Ed., 186–206, Sage, Los Angeles, 1989.
22. Krippner, S., A questionnaire study of experiential reactions to a Brazilian healer, *J. Soc. Psychical Res.*, 56, 208–215, 1990.

23. Krippner, S., Cross-cultural perspectives on hypnotic-like procedures used by native healing practitioners, in *Handbook of Clinical Hypnosis*, J.W. Rhue, S.J. Lynn, and I. Kirsch, Eds., 691–717, American Psychological Assoc., Washington, D.C., 1993.

24. Kroger, W.S., *Clinical and Experimental Hypnosis*, 2nd ed., Lippincott, Philadelphia, 1977.

25. Leacock, S. and Leacock, R., *Spirits of the Deep: drums, mediums and trance in a Brazilian city*, Doubleday, Garden City, New York, 1972.

26. Lynn, S.L. and Rhue, J., Fantasy proneness: hypnosis, developmental antecedents, and psychopathology, *Am. Psycholog.*, 43, 35–44, 1988.

27. Murphy, G., *Personality: a biosocial approach to origins and structure*, Harper and Brothers, New York, 1947.

28. Price-Williams, D., *Explorations in cross-cultural psychology*, Chandler and Sharp, San Francisco, 1975.

29. Raboteau, A.J., The Afro-American traditions, in *Caring and curing: Health and medicine in Western religious traditions*, R.L. Numbers and D.W. Amundsen, Eds., 539–562, Macmillan, New York, 1986.

30. Richeport, M.M., The interface between multiple personality, spirit mediumship, and hypnosis, *Am. J. Clin. Hypnosis*, 34, 168–177, 1992.

31. Rogers, S.L., *The Shaman: his symbols and his healing power*, Charles Thomas, Springfield, IL, 1982.

32. Sandner, D., *Navaho Symbols of Healing*, Harcourt Brace Jovanovich, New York, 1979.

33. Spanos, N.P., Hypnosis, demonic possession, and multiple personality: strategic enactments and disavowals of responsibility for actions, in *Altered States of Consciousness and Mental Health: a cross-cultural perspective*, C. Ward, Ed., 96–124, Los Angeles, Sage, 1989.

34. Strupp, H.H., On the technology of psychotherapy, *Arch. Gen. Psychiatr.*, 26, 270–278, 1989.

35. Suryani, L.K. and Jensen, G.D., *Trance and possession in Bali: a window on Western multiple personality*, Oxford University Press, New York, 1993.

36. Thong, D., with Carpenter, B. and Krippner, S., *A Psychiatrist in Paradise: treating mental illness in Bali*, White Lotus Press, Bangkok, Thailand, 1994.

37. Topper, M.D., The traditional Navajo medicine man: therapist, counselor, and community leader, *J. Psychoanalytic Anthropol.*, 10, 217–249, 1987.

38. Torrey, E.F., *Witchdoctors and Psychiatrists: the common roots of psychotherapy and its future*, Harper & Row, New York, 1986.

39. Vogel, V.J., *American Indian medicine*, University of Oklahoma Press, Norman, OK, 1990.

40. Walsh, R., and Vaughan, F., Introduction, In *Beyond ego: Transpersonal dimensions in psychology*, R. Walsh and F. Vaughan Eds., 15–24, J.P. Tarcher, Los Angeles, 1980.

41. Winkelman, M., A cross-cultural study of magico-religious practitioners, in *Proc. Int. Conf. Shamanism*, R.-I. Heinze, Ed., 27–38, Independent Scholars of Asia, Berkeley, 1984.

For further study:

Center for Shamanic Studies
Contact Michael Harner, Ph.D.
P.O. Box 1939
Mill Valley, CA 94942

Independent Scholars of Asia
Contact Ruth-Inge Heinze, Ph.D.
Suite 3-C, 2321 Russell Street
Berkeley, CA 95705

chapter thirteen

Channeling and hypnosis

Eric D. Leskowitz

Introduction

Imagine the dilemma of poor Jeremiah, the son of an Israelite priest living in pastoral Judea in 1200 B.C., who reported the following experience in 1:4-10:

> The word of the Lord came to me: "Before I created you in the womb, I selected you; before you were born, I consecrated you; I appointed you a prophet concerning the nations." I replied: "Ah, Lord God! I don't know how to speak, for I am still a boy". And the Lord said to me: "Do not say, 'I am still a boy', but go wherever I send you and speak whatever I command you. Have no fear of them, for I am with you to deliver you."

> The Lord put out His hand and touched my mouth, and the Lord said to me: "Herewith I put My words into your mouth. See, I appoint you this day over nations and kingdoms; to uproot and to pull down, to destroy and to overthrow, to build and to plant."

First psychotic break, or mystical experience? The auditory hallucinations of schizophrenia, or a deep spiritual insight delivered by the mechanism of channeling? This differential diagnosis is crucial to the discussion in this chapter, because an entire source of valuable metaphysical information can too easily be dismissed if the process for obtaining it is pathologized. Our Western culture tends to dismiss paranormal experiences like prophecy as the result of psychopathology, the short-circuiting of a broken brain. St. Paul's conversion experience on the road to Damascus has been explained as simply an epileptic seizure, while Joan of Arc was said to suffer manic delusions of grandeur.[1] And yet despite the medical community's disdain, the words and deeds of these people have had the power to move thousands (unlike the ineffective and chaotic words and deeds of the truly delusional or brain disordered).

Our modern materialist worldview has no room for transpersonal experiences. In today's secular America, one could imagine Jeremiah disrupting his quiet suburban neighborhood with his harsh words, and then being quickly committed to the local psychiatric hospital. After "rapid neurolepti-zation" via Haldol, there would follow a quick discharge back into the community a few days later, due to limited HMO coverage for psychiatric care. And then he'd be lost to follow up, his insights and warnings muffled by his psychotropic medications, perhaps breaking through again later as part of the "revolving door" syndrome that plagues inpatient psychiatric treatment. But the tide may be turning; for example, Neal Walsch's *Conversations with God*, a modern version of Jeremiah's experience, has been a recent bestseller.

Fortunately for Jeremiah (and for the Israelites), his Old Testament culture was quite comfortable with the notion that God could speak directly to man. Those men chosen to be intermediaries with God were esteemed in their culture, and were called prophets. In other words, the propehts did the same work that had been done at other times and in other cultures by mediums or oracles or shamans.[2] The Israelites were not the only people to believe in prophecy; consider the classical Greeks during their Golden Age. Their poets and playwrights awaited the inspiration of their muses, not just metaphors for the process of inspiration, but conscious living entities with whom some artists were privileged to have a direct relationship. For the masses, there were the oracles at Delphi, Pythia, and elsewhere. Priests would act as intermediaries to the world of spirit and relay direct communications to interested humans. Therefore it seems that two of the primary sources for modern Western or Judeo-Christian civilization held mediumship or channeling (two terms for the same process) to be their most important source of spiritual insights.

Similarly, the founders of most religions claim to speak the word of God directly. Jesus repeatedly makes this claim, and Mohammed states that the Koran was dictated directly to him while in an extended state of spiritual ecstasy. Even European high culture from the Renaissance onward has paid heed to courting the muse, from Shakespeare to the Impressionists, from Bach and Mozart (both of whom believed they were transcribing angelic choirs) to Rodin. By contrast, something seems to have happened in our post-Industrial, 20th century information age which devalues and pathologizes inspiration. The sociological aspects of this transitional phenomenon are discussed in more detail by Price-Williams,[3] and Krippner (in Chapter 12 of this book).

Chapter overview

In this chapter, the perspective of transpersonal psychology will be brought to bear on the trance process known as channeling, the modern version of courting the muse or Biblical prophecy. I will look at some recent psychological studies of the process of channeling, especially at comparisons with such superficially similar trance states as dissociation and multiple personality disorder. The uniqueness of channeling, and the psychological health of the practitioner, will become evident. I will also provide two extensive excerpts of material delivered by modern channels, and ask the readers to assess for themselves the validity and utility of this material.

Of course, the key aspect of channeling that skeptics focus on is the validity of the information that is brought to us through this process. Since scientific validation comes so readily for externalized, objective, physical phenomena, measurement of the physiological changes which accompany the process of channeling have been pursued. These studies are fascinating and provide important correlations, but they are still inadequate to answer questions of validity.

Psychophysiology cannot answer questions of validity because our technology is too coarse to measure and answer metaphysical issues. We can only detect the effects of these processes on human physiology. So instead of trying to "prove" the validity of the process by presenting some objective experimentation, I will simply follow the research summary with several channeled documents that I have personally found useful in understanding how the universe operates. I ask readers to use their own internal discernment to assess these thoughts. Consider them as opinions, use them if they work for you, and discard them if they don't.

According to a widely held view about prophecy, we can simply wait and see whether the predictions come true; if they do not materialize, then the prophecy is clearly wrong. However, this simple viewpoint ignores the "advance warning" aspect of prophecy. Many of these messages about future disaster are supposedly brought to human attention in the hopes that the free will actions of the people will help avert the predicted catastrophe. Thus, if a prediction does not materialize as it was foretold, it can be argued that the prediction was in fact successful; it alerted people enough to change their course of action and avert the disaster. In the realm of objective validation of prophecy, it seems, there is no easy answer.

Psychophysiology of channeling

To highlight some current correlational studies of trance channeling, we turn to the work of psychologist Dureen Hughes. She has studied both psychophysiological and psychological aspects of the channelling process, and has outlined in some detail the key phenomenologic aspects of this process.[4] She has also compared channelling to such pathological states as multiple personality disorder (MPD, though it's now more accurately called dissociative identity disorder, or DID) and dissociation,[5] using standardized psychodiagnostic intstruments.

To review, dissociation is the psychological defense mechanism which protects us from overwhelming anxiety by splitting our awareness away from the anxiety of a traumatic moment; it creates a sense of unreality, distance, and distorted time. It is a common aspect of post-traumatic stress disorder (PTSD); the nightmares and flashbacks of this syndrome represent emotionally charged material breaking through the barrier of dissociation, back into conscious awareness. Dissociation occurs in degrees of intensity, and there is a spectrum of dissociative symptoms that range from common "highway hypnosis" (driving succesfully to your destination despite daydreaming the entire time), through PTSD flashbacks (wherein the past becomes more real than the present), to MPD (where consciousness is so divided that separate selves seem to coexist within one being). Hypnosis has come to be regarded as an essential therapeutic tool in treating PTSD, because it helps the patient control his own dissociative process through a form of self-directed dissociation.[6]

Hughes' studies have compared MPD to channeling because both phenomena are characterized by apparently shared consciousnesses within one host being. In other words, Hughes is asking whether the "spirit guide" is simply a part of the host channeler's personality, traumatically split off into an alter personality's voice, or an independent conscious entity. If channeling were merely an exotic form of psychopathology, or a less stigmatizing presentation of MPD, then one would expect to see many of the other symptoms of major dissociative disorders in channelers. Importantly, Hughes found[5] that her cohort of 10 channelers reported far fewer dissociative experiences than did typical MPD patients, and in fact scored well within the normal range on several clinical measures of dissociative tendences (including the DES, the Dissociative Experiences Scale). Channelers also lacked the antecedent history of childhood abuse typically experienced by MPD patients. Further, the unusual split in awareness that occured during their channeling sessions happened under their conscious control, unlike the unpredictable dissociative response to stress that characterizes MPD. Thus, there was no significant psychopathology evident in the channellers, as predicted by the MPD hypothesis.

Physiologically, EEG brainwave patterns were measured before, during, and after channeling sessions.[7] Statistically significant changes were noted, with increased time of cortical alpha wave activity resulting. The localization of these frequency changes to different areas of the cortex was unfortunately not studied, and so any specific regional changes were lost in these global measures. Similar findings of predominant alpha wave activity have been documented in hypnotic trance.[8] Hopefully, research can be done to study specific patterns of brain activation (via SPECT and PET scans, etc.) during channeling, as is now being done by Shin and van der Kolk during PTSD dissociations,[9] to understand what brain mechanisms mediate this process. However, unlike the reductionistic models of PTSD which look to the amygdala, for example, as the causal locus of PTSD symptoms, a transpersonal view of trance channeling would hold that activation in the amygdala (or any "hot spots" in the brain that are found) occurs because this is the site where high frequency spiritual energy input is "stepped down," or transduced, into the vibrational range of physiologic processes. This frequency model was described in more detail in Chapter 3 of this book.

Energetic aspects of channeling

Another method of detecting specific changes that occur during these various trance experiences has not been fully validated technologically, but still provides intriguing phenomenological data that helps answer the question of what happens during trance channeling. As described earlier in Chapter 2, many people have demonstrated a reliable ability to detect changes in the human energy field (see Reference 10 for a well-controlled study). Given the potential validity of the energy field model described throughout this book, it should be possible for medical clairvoyants to detect changes in energy fields of subjects who channel. These changes could then be compared and contrasted to the changes that occur when a subject undergoes a simple hypnotic induction.

A formal experimental protocol for this type of research has not yet been devised, but informal conversations with several medical clairvoyants who also have graduate training in the health sciences show a consistent pattern. That is, the energy field of a channeler is uniformly described as becoming brighter, more focused and more "high frequency" when the entity begins to transmit information. Often there is a perception that the etheric form (or subtle body) of the spiritual being somehow overlies or intertwines with the channeler's human body, so as to animate it on a physical level. Witnesses describe changes in mannerism, physical habitus, speech patterns and regional accent, as well as changes in clarity of thought and depth of wisdom, attendant with the onset of the transmission.

In simple hypnosis, i.e., guided imagery for relaxation, there is a clairvoyant perception of the energy field calming, with a brightness or focus in the forehead region; the third eye seems to get activated, and the internal images themselves sometimes become visible in the energy body. However, there are no massive overall transformations in the nature of the host field itself, certainly not to the degree described during observations of channeling sessions.

Those are some lines of evidence that suggest that channeling is not the result of psychopathology, but may instead actually represent a heightened activation and receptivity of the human nervous system during a unique type of transpersonal trance. In the final section of this chapter, I will present some samples of channeled information, without editorial comment, leaving the reader to decide its validity.

Channeled information: the Seth material

The first source, Jane Roberts, began her career as an art teacher in upstate New York and began to experiment in ESP with her husband in the mid-1960s. Very quickly, Roberts began to receive thought impressions from a personality who identified himself as "Seth." Roberts found it easiest to transmit this information by allowing "him" to speak out loud, using her voice. The result was a series of 15 books written over the next 25 years, until Roberts' death in 1986. The books have sold over 5 million copies worldwide and are often credited with sparking the current revival of interest in channeled information.[11]

Seth cryptically described himself as "an energy personality essence no longer focused in physical reality" and used his transpersonal perspective to provide a vast amount of information on many diverse topics. Consider the following chapter titles from several of his/her books: "The Physical Universe as Idea Construction," "Dreamtime Bleed-Throughs of Reincarnational Memory," "The Physical Body as a Living Sculpture," and "Group Dreams and the Formation of Mass Events."

Perhaps Seth's most quoted (and misinterpreted) statement was, "You create your own reality." Oft quoted because of the sense of empowerment it conveyed, misinterpreted because of the blaming mentality that became attached to it, i.e., "Why did you create that lung cancer?" The subtlety of this multidimensional concept escapes those who seek an easy target for frustration and blame, and who try to dismiss holistic medicine categorically. The way to understand this slogan clearly is to remember the important distinction between the "I" who creates the reality (the higher self or transpersonal agent) vs. the "I" who experiences daily life (the less than fully conscious personality level self). The higher self creates the reality of the personal ego, with which most of us identify.

To help appreciate the richness behind this slogan, I have selected several excerpts from Roberts' book *The Nature of Personal Reality*, from the chapters entitled: "Natural Hypnosis: a trance is a trance is a trance," and "Natural Hypnosis, Healing, and the Transference of Physical Symptoms to Other Levels of Activity." They were chosen because they place the hypnotic process in the larger context of transpersonal dimensions. At the same time, I hope that these excerpts will normalize and humanize the otherwise grandiose sounding process of trance channeling.

The first part of Seth's discourse defines natural hypnosis as the way we focus on our own hidden beliefs through continual self-dialogue. It is a good explanation of simple clinical hypnosis, as well:

> Natural hypnosis is the acquiescence of the unconscious to conscious belief. In periods of concentrated focus, with all distractions cut the desired ideas are then implanted (in formal hypnosis). The same processes occur in normal life, however; areas of primary concentration then regulate your experience both biologically and mentally, and generate similar conditions ... Your beliefs, then, are like hypnotic focuses. You reinforce them constantly through the normal inner talking in which you all indulge.

This inner communication acts like the constant repetition of a hypnotist. In this case, however, you are your
own hypnotist. ... You can perform physical feats that
you would consider impossible otherwise — all of this
because you willingly suspend certain beliefs and allow yourself to accept others for the moment. Unfortunately, because of the patter considered necessary, it
is thought that the conscious mind is lulled and its
activity suspended. Quite the contrary. It is focused,
intensified, narrowed to a specific area, and all other
stimuli are cut out.

This intensity of conscious concentration cuts down
barriers and allows the messages to go directly to the
unconscious, where they are acted upon. The hypnotist, however, *is* important in that he acts as a direct
representative of authority.

Consider now some of Seth's thoughts on the "primitive" transcultural
trance of witch doctors (see Krippner in Chapter 12 of this book for a full
exposition of indigenous trance):

In your terms, beliefs are accepted initially from the
parents — this, as mentioned earlier, having to do with
mammalian experience. The hypnotist then acts as a
parent substitute. In cases of therapy, an individual is
already frightened, and because of the beliefs in your
civilization, he looks not to himself but to an authority
figure for help. Even in primitive societies, witch doctors and other natural therapists have understood that
the point of power is in the present, and they have
utilized natural hypnosis as a method of helping other
individuals to concentrate their own energy. All of the
gestures, dances, and other procedures are shock treatment, startling the subject out of habitual reactions so
that he or she is forced to focus upon the present moment. The resulting disorientation simply shakes current beliefs and dislodges set frameworks. The
hypnotist, or witch doctor, or therapist, then immediately inserts the beliefs he thinks the subject needs.

Seth then looks at the limiting beliefs of modern hypnotherapists and
physicians (yes, even doctors have limiting beliefs):

Within this context, subsidiary groupings (of beliefs -
Ed.) will be included that involve the therapist's own

ideas. In your society, regression is often involved; the
patient will remember and relive a traumatic experience
from the past. This will then appear to be the cause of
the present difficulty. If the hypnotist and the subject
both accept this (belief - Ed.), then at that level there will
be progress. If the cultural concepts include voodoo or
witchcraft, then the therapeutic situation will be seen in
that context, and a cure uncovered; which, using the
power point of the present, the doctor will then reverse.

Quite without the context of formal hypnosis, however, the same issues apply. With the greatest understanding and compassion, let be mention that Western
medicine is in its way one of the most uncivilized
hypnotic devices. The most educated Western doctors
will look with utter dismay and horror at the thought
of a chicken being sacrificed in a primitive witch doctor's hut, and yet will consider it quite scientific and
inevitable that a woman sacrifice two breasts to cancer.
The doctors will simply see no other way out, and
unfortunately neither will the patient.

A modern Western physician — granted, with the
greatest discomfiture — will inform his patient that he
is about to die, impressing upon him that his situation
is hopeless, and yet will react with scorn and loathing
when he reads that a voodoo practitioner has put a
curse upon some innocent victim.

In your time, medical men, again with great superiority,
look at primitive cultures and harshly judge the villag-
ers they think are held in the sway of witch doctors or
voodooism; and yet through advertisement and organization, *your* doctors impress upon each individual in
your culture that you must have a physical examination
every six months or you will get cancer; that you must
have medical insurance because you *will* become ill.

In many instances, therefore, modern physicians are
inadequate witch doctors who have forgotten their
craft — hypnotists who no longer believe in the power
of healing, and whose suggestions bring about other
diseases which are diagnosed in advance.

You are told what to look for; you are as cursed — far
more — as any native in a tiny village, only you lose

breasts, appendixes, and other portions of your anatomy. The doctors follow their own ideas, of course, and in that system they see themselves as completely justified — as humane.

In the medical field, as in no other, you are faced directly with the full impact of your beliefs, for the doctors are not the healthiest, but the least healthy. They fall prey to the beliefs to which they so heartily subscribe. Their concentration is upon disease, not health.

Here are Seth's thoughts about health insurance and the fear of illness:

You are paying in advance for illness that you are certain will come your way. You are making all preparations in the present for a future of illness. You are betting upon disease and not health. This is the worst kind of natural hypnosis, and yet within your system, insurance is indeed a necessity because the belief in illness so pervades your mental atmosphere.

Many become ill only *after* taking out such "insurance" — and for those, the act itself symbolically represents an acceptance of disease. Even more unfortunate are the special policies for the elderly that detail in advance all of the most stereotyped and distorted concepts about health and age. There is a great correlation between the kind of policies that people take out, and the illnesses that they fall prey to.

Generally speaking, those who advocate health foods or natural foods subscribe to some of the same overall beliefs held by your physicians. They believe that diseases are the result of exterior conditions.

Moral values become attached to food, with some seen as good and some as bad. Symptoms appear, and are quite directly considered to be the natural result of ingesting foods on the forbidden list. You are what you *think,* not what you eat — and to a large extent what you *think* about what you eat is far more important. ... The best diet in the world, by *anyone's* standards, will not keep you healthy if you have a belief in illness.

Your thoughts are reality. They directly affect your body. It seems that you are highly civilized people because you put your ill into hospitals where they can be cared for.

What you do, of course, is to isolate a group of people who are filled with negative beliefs about illness. The contagion of beliefs spreads. Patients are obviously in hospitals *because they are ill*. The sick and their doctors both work on that principle.

Women delivering children are placed in the same environment. This may seem very humane to you, and yet the entire system is structured so that childbirth does not seem to be the result of health but of illness.

Stimuli pertaining to health are effectively blocked in such organizations. The ill are gathered together and denied all of their normal and natural conditions, including the compensating motivations that *alone* would sometimes be enough to *restore health* if given time.

Your beliefs then are highly important in the way in which you handle the power of personal action.

The use of your private energy brings you into intimate relationship with your own source of power. Healing involves great natural aggressive thrusts of energy, growth and the focus of vitality. The more powerless you feel, the less able you are to utilize your own healing abilities. You are then forced to project these outward upon a physician, a healer, or any outside agency. If your own belief in the physician "works," and you are cured of symptoms, you are physically relieved, and yet your own belief in yourself may be further infringed upon. If you are making no effective efforts to handle your own problems, then the symptoms will simply reappear in a new fashion, and the same process will be reinitiated. You may lose faith in your doctor while still retaining confidence in doctors as a whole, and run from one to another.

But the body has its own integrity, and illness is often simply a natural sign of imbalance, a physical message to which you are to listen and make inner adjustments accordingly.

When these realignments are always made from the outside, the body's innate coherence becomes jeopardized, and its intimate relationship with mind is confused. More, its natural healing powers are *dulled*. The built-in initiating riggers of reactions that are meant to follow inner stimuli are activated instead by "exterior" means.

The individual's faith is transferred more and more to an outside agency. This usually means that no time is allowed for necessary inner dialogues or self-questioning, and the self-healing that might otherwise occur is brought about through belief in another.

The point of power, again, is in the present, when your nonphysical self merges with corporeal reality. The recognition of that fact alone can revitalize your life.

In your terms, you are in a state of evolution as a species. Part of this experience includes a natural fascination with exterior events. You are developing properties of consciousness that are in their own way uniquely your own, as your environment is. A strong focus is a necessary counterpart, since you are involved in a learning process in which all elements inherent in the situation will be explored.

Throughout this venture, however, you are in the dream state, always kept in touch with the realities from which your physical experience springs. As you understand time, you will eventually be able to merge your inner comprehension with your physical self, and form your world on a conscious basis. Such manuscripts as mine are meant to help you do precisely that."

A brief commentary is in order, particularly regarding the previously mentioned argument over who creates our reality. Seth shows that by focusing intently on the present moment, his so-called "point of power," we are able to bring untold energies from transpersonal realms to bear on changing our limited but palpable physical reality. He does not intend to blame people for their life dilemmas (as critics of New Age thinking allege) because that would simply perpetuate the victim mentality that these teachings were explicitly designed to overcome. Instead, it may be most helpful to view this Sethian excerpt as an example of the unconscious ways in which we can hypnotically program ourselves to experience life in one certain way and to thereby unwittingly create external situations to match our hidden expectations and needs. The emphasis in the Seth books in the References at the end of this chapter is on those transpersonal parts of ourselves, the higher self, the soul, that do create life situations (including seemingly arbitrary ones like birth status, life tasks, and personal aptitudes), even when our conscious personality or egoic mind is largely oblivious to the process.

A channeled explanation of channeling

Before turning to another even more exotic source of channeled information, I will say something about the energetic dynamics of the channeling process as a way of better understanding the actual mechanism by which this phenomenon occurs. I begin with a quotation from the source known as Alexander (whose channel, a writer named Ramon Stevens, types down, rather than speaks aloud, his information[12]):

> What occurs in the trance state between you (Ramon
> - Ed.)) and me (Alexander - Ed.) is that we construct a
> psychological bridge between our realities. You send
> up a vibrational frequency that meets with mine, vi-
> brating at a higher frequency; together our differing
> frequencies create a third, unique energy field which
> you can think of as a psychological bridge. Our infor-
> mation (Alexander is a collective consciousness, hence
> the plural pronoun - Ed.) is assembled in nonphysical,
> nonspoken form; we then send it down across that
> psychological bridge, and it is at this point that the
> original intent of the material is translated into English.
> Your vocabulary is employed, and the grids of intent
> behind our ideas riffle through your vocabulary as in
> a dictionary, searching out the precise meaning. Once
> a grid of intent finds appropriate language to give it
> expression, it drops out of the psychological bridge
> into your energy field, where it is transmitted through
> your neuronal structure into the physical act of typing
> on the keyboard.

Even after this psychological bridge has been constructed, accurate channeling requires extreme emotional clarity on the part of the medium. Discordant emotional energy distorts the information being received. A coherent, synchronous, high frequency energy field is thus needed in order to accurately channel information; accordingly, many well-known trance teachers hold their sessions in a group setting. This coherent group is all on the same energetic wavelength and is able to hold the stable high intensity energy field that allows the channel to reach up and create that stable psychological bridge to the even more highly refined energy of the teaching entity.

The channel's filters can become colored by any significant personal emotional biases he or she may have, as well as biases among his/her audience. Furthermore, repeated exposure of the channel over time to the transformative energies of spirit teachers, without consistent emotional clearing work, can lead to the surfacing of significant distortions. As these distortions creep in, the channeled messages gradually lose the clarity and majesty which initially attracted the followers. The channel can then become a mirror for the group's unconscious beliefs, via a sort of energetic projective identification (as psychoanalysts might call it), rather than a clear transmitter of valuable new information.

This is one possible explanation for the lengthy melodrama involving one of the most publicized Californian channels, J. Z. Knight, and her spirit guide Ramtha. Lawsuits over the issue of Ms. Knight's personal legal responsiblity for the accuracy of Ramtha's messages and instructions have left her spiritual community in shambles; novel legal doctrines regarding personal responsibility for the messages of a spirit guide have arisen. Perhaps the glare of celebrity and glamour shifted the focus off spiritual teachings. But this and other related New Age events have engendered criticism. For example, the cartoon strip "Doonesbury" portrays the starlet character "Boopsie" spontaneously channeling "Hunk-Ra," a 40,000 year old warrior whose ludicrous teachings have effectively discredited the phenomenon of channeling for many readers of Doonesbury. In other words, channeling can be similar to playing with fire — a certain amount of training protects against being burned. To that end, the references after this chapter include information on several reliable training programs in mediumship in America today.

Non-terrestrial sources of information

This chapter will now move to some information channeled from what is best described as a nonterrestrial source. For if we follow the logic implicit in this entire book, that awareness is not dependent on the human brain for its existence, then it should not be surprising to consider that awarenesses may exist which do not take a human form and which do not even need to physically focus on Earth in order to carry on their life purpose. I am not talking about animal consciousness and its transpersonal dimension (see the work of animal communicator Penelope Smith[13] for a discussion of this phenomenon). Rather, I am talking about extraterrestrial intelligence. Obviously this is a controversial notion. I hope you'll find it provocative, even if you do decide to read it as science fiction rather than as clinical psychology.

Our ongoing cultural evaluation of the question of extraterrestrial beings is highly tainted by media sensationalism even when it is skillfully presented, as in television programs such as "The X-Files." This is, after all, a phenomenon that deserves scientific inquiry, even if only to understand the reason for the persistence of mass delusions. The work of John Mack, the Harvard psychiatrist who wrote *Abductions*,[14] brings this a spirit of scientific investigation to this controversial field. His work focused on the so-called abduction phenomenon, wherein non-benign extraterrestrials (ET) are supposed to manipulate Earthlings for their own benefit, rather than to guide us into higher knowledge as an aid to our human evolution.

Not surprisingly, other species of ET exist which are believed to have a more benign intent towards humanity. Several books are now available which contain channeled material purportedly coming from these more helpful ETs. *Bringers of the Dawn*[15] is accessible to newcomers to the field and outlines a "Star Trek"-like storyline for events currently unfolding in today's world; *The Starseed Transmissions*[16] is a majestic presentation of a similar scenario for human transformation. Parenthetically, the creator of "Star Trek," Gene Roddenberry, was involved in channeling experiments and his vision of intergalactic cooperation may have been inspired by some of his direct personal experiences of allegedly nonterrestrial intelligence.[17]

More and more people are now learning to access these off-planet sources of information; one such person is a licensed clinical social worker in the Boston area. Although she prefers to remain anonymous, she has kindly devoted time to allowing the entities who claim to represent the Pleiades star cluster in the constellation Taurus (and known to Native Americans as the Seven Sisters) to speak through her. The following information is excerpted from a recent conversation with her/them. By way of background, this channel's skills developed over the course of three years of intense psychic work in a group format. She initially experienced an involuntary and somewhat frightening urge to make wordless sounds, but now she simply closes her eyes and becomes quiet for about 15 seconds. She then begins to speak in a voice quite like her everyday voice, betraying no unusual accent; yet it has a depth and clarity which she herself will admit she does not possess (even on her best days).

The question I asked her was, "Could you please comment on the use of hypnosis to access multidimensional states?" The answer that follows has been lightly edited, to smooth out the often cumbersome grammar used by her spirit friend:

> Hypnosis is simply a tiny, tiny speck of your capacity for transversing multidimensionally. If you were to fuel a car with it, it would not go very far. It is, however, manageable in your dimension, and so in its manageability many find it a useful tool. It is similar to a hand-held can opener, useful and yet somewhat jagged and awkward. Some, as they reach within the can that has been opened, cut their hand on the jagged edges, and thus many recoil from its use. It is not that it is not useful, it is simply that it is often jagged and difficult in its manageability. And yet for many the can is opened and nourishment is available, and they are pleased by that, and so they stop going to the market.

To only eat canned goods, and to need to do that carefully, is somewhat limiting.

But ask more specifically - there are things that run
and race through your mind, and we enjoy our visit.

I asked, "Can you say something about the relationship between trance
and energy field states?"

As the being uses the can opener to open the can, there
is for that being a hope of being fed. And so the can
is opened and often there is disappointment in the
contents that appear in the can. Sometimes, even
though there is disappointment, if there is need, there
is feeding. Sometimes there is such need that in the
entering of the hand into the can, there is damage and
tearing. Within the being, fear is created. And so, often
at that moment there is a closing down of the being
from those areas that might have been accessed, had
there been a willingness to move forewared into a careful monitoring and emptying of the can. Trance itself,
as we have said, is quite limited in its capacity to
nourish and feed the beings of your dimension. Useful, but narrow and limited.

The concept of energetic forms ("energy field states" -
Ed.), while somewhat broader, is also quite limited.
Energetic forms - and we understand that they are dear
to the hearts of you and the one who speaks (i.e., the
channel - Ed.) - are, we feel, at your current stage,
simply a better can opener. You use it, you use it with
ease and expediency, you plug it into an energetic
source, it opens the rim without the jagged edges,
many are able to dip in and out, without the damage
that occurs with the earlier form of this tool, and yet
it is still simply a particular tool that is used to open
a very limited source of nourishment.

You will notice as you move from that which is jagged
and hand-held to that which is smoother and plugged
into a source of current, that you find more and more
possibilities - larger cans, smaller cans, things held in
these cans that are different. And that is pleasant. It is
our request that you not be so captivated by the capacity to nourish yourself with canned goods that you
forget to go to the market! There is in the universe a

much broader field of nourishment than you currently understand. As you continue to be open to explore that, heed well our advice to move into areas different from what you currently believe and know to be true. For while your belief and knowledge is not inaccurate, it is still quite limited; and in holding to it too dearly, you will limit yourselves.

I guess we humans are finally getting ready to make the transition from canned food to fresh food (organically grown, no doubt) — in other words, our energetic metabolism is evolving to the point where we can handle direct contact with unprocessed sources of spiritual energy. And transpersonal hypnosis is apparently just a very primitive way to access this cosmic food at least from a Pleiadian perspective.

Conclusion

Nevertheless, as we begin to sample from the veritable smorgasbord of channeled meals now being offered up to us, we would do well to heed the advice of Alexander, in my opinion the most earthly and most humorous spirit guide now in print. He describes how Western civilization's divorce from nature and divinity is leading to a collapse of our society's major institutions, at the same time that many of its citizens are being drawn toward radically new ways of thinking and acting, towards what he calls the new order:

> The phenomenon of channeling occurs because you are so desperate for knowledge as to how to right your course that those straddling new and old orders can indeed serve as channels for discarnate information. But once the new order is established, channeling will cease. You will channel nature. You will channel yourselves, if you can excuse the imagery. This is why channeling is rising in incidence at this time and will continue to do so until the establishment of a new order. Your psyches are being yanked in two directions; the species cries out for guidance, and it is part of our growth to provide what we can.

> Let us just affirm that you are a divine creature, that you are rooted in a natural order of absolute security and that there is nothing to fear. The only harm that can come to you is when you allow it to come to you by abdicating your reason and your intrinsic sense of your own divinity and your own worth. Don't let feelings of

responsiblity stop you from enjoying your life, from
pursuing those avenues of pleasure which give your life
enrichment. Don't think that you have to save the world.
You will automatically help save the world just by being
yourself and by being happy with who you are. The
happiness comes first; the rest follows.[12]

To which I can only add, Amen!

References

1. Blumer, Dietrich, The Psychiatric Dimension of Epilepsy: historical perspective and current significance, in *Psychiatric Aspects of Epilepsy*, Dietrich Blumer, Ed., APA Press, Washington D.C., 1984.
2. Klimo, Jon, *Psychics, Prophets and Mystics: receiving information from paranormal sources*, The Aquarian Press/Harper Collins Publishers, London, UK, 1991.
3. Price-Williams, D. and Hughes, D., Shamanism and Altered States of Consciousness, *Anthropology of Consciousness*, 5:2, 1–15, 1994.
4. Hughes, D., Blending with an Other: an analysis of trance channeling in the United States, *Ethos*, 19(2), 161–184, 1991.
5. Hughes, D., Differences Between Trance Channeling and Multiple Personality Disorder on Structured Interview, *J. Transpersonal Psychol.*, 24:2, 181–192, 1992.
6. Smith, W. H., Incorporating hypnosis into the psychotherapy of patients with multiple personality disorder, *Bulletin of the Menninger Clinics*, 57(3):344-354, 1993.
7. Hughes, D. and Melville, N., Changes in Brainwave Activity During Trance Channeling: a pilot study, *J. Transpersonal Psychol.*, 22:2, 175–189, 1990.
8. Graffin, et al., EEG Concomitants of Hypnosis and Hypnotic Susceptibility, *J. Abnormal Psychol.*, 104(1):123–131, 1995.
9. Shin, Bessel, and van de Kolk, Visual Imagery and Perception in Posttraumatic Stress Disorder: a positron emission tomographic investigation, *Archives of General Psychiatry*, 54:233–241, 1997.
10. Hunt, Valerie, The Rolf Study, *Wheels of Light: chakras, auras, and the healing energy of the body*, Appendix 1 in Bruyere, Rosalyn, Fireside Books, New York, 1994.
11. Roberts, Jane, *The Nature of Personal Reality*, Prentice Hall Books, New York, 1974. See also: by Roberts *Seth Speaks*, 1972, *The Education of Oversoul Seven*, 1973, and *The Nature of the Psyche: Its Human Expression*, 1979.
12. Stevens, Ramon, *Whatever Happened to Divine Grace?*, Stillpoint Press, Walpole, N.H., 1988.
13. Smith, Penelope, *Animals: our return to wholeness*, Pegasus Publications, Point Reyes, CA, 1993.
14. Mack, John, *Abduction*, 1995.
15. Marciniak, Barbara, *Bringers of the Dawn*, Bear and Co., Santa Fe, 1992.
16. Carey, Ken, *The Starseed Transmissions*, Harper, San Francisco, 1991.
17. Schlemmer, Phyllis and Jenkins, Palden, in *The Universal Civilizations*, *The Only Planet of Choice*, Gateway Books, Bath, UK, 1993, chap. 6.

For further study:

Barbara Brennan School of Healing
PO Box 2005
East Hampton, NY 11937
(516) 329-0951
http://www.barbarabrennan.com

Healing Light Center Church
PO Box 758
Sierra Madre, CA 91025
(818) 306-2170

Lily Dale Assembly
5 Melrose Park Suite J
Lily Dale, NY 14752
(716) 595-2442

INDEX